Growth Mindset

Destroy your Fears, Build the Mindset Toughness of the True Warrior thanks to the New Psychology of Success!

Written by C. Baker

Table of Contents

Chapter 1. Introduction

Chapter 2. What Is Your Why?

Chapter 3. Fighting The Curse of Unrealistic Expectations

Chapter 4. A Warrior Keeps His Promises

Chapter 5. Sharpen Your Sword

- 3 tasks a day
- Doing just enough to be a little uncomfortable
- Do the most difficult task first
- Activity and work are two different things
- Know when to take a break

Chapter 6. The Importance of Focus

Chapter 7. Battling The Fear Demons

1. Fear of the Unknown
2. The Fear of Failure
3. The Fear That You Are Not Good Enough
4. The Fear That You're Late or Too Old
5. Limiting Beliefs

Chapter 8. Climb The Staircase That You Can't See

- Visualize your success
- Prayer is powerful
- Read autobiographies of successful people
- Motivate yourself regularly

Chapter 9. A Tiger Doesn't Lose Sleep Over The Opinions Of Sheep

- Look at your why
- Remember the bamboo tree
- Get motivated
- Know that it's all turbulence
- Success turns naysayers into supporters
- Understand the psychology behind it

Chapter 10. Weight Loss Is Simpler Than You Think

1. Cut the carbs
2. Intermittent fasting
3. Get enough sleep
4. Fasted cardio
5. Shorter but higher intensity workouts
6. Eat Foods That Burn Fat
7. Drink Lots of Water
8. Have a Food Journal

Chapter 11. From Ideal Weight To A Six Pack

Chapter 12. Calories

Chapter 13. Training

Chapter 14. Diet

Chapter 15. Building Muscle and Gaining Mass

Chapter 16. How many reps and sets?

Chapter 17. How much muscle can I hope to gain?

Chapter 18. Before you start with weights.

Chapter 19. Don't neglect your posture and flexibility

Chapter 20. A Warrior Watches His Money

- What's your number?
- Money is oxygen to your business
- Can you do both effectively
- Your six-month nest egg
- Insurance and medical benefits
- Is your spouse working?

Chapter 21. The Biggest Secret To Making Money Online

Chapter 22. What's shiny object syndrome?

- Most of it is noise
- Focus on just one method
- Stick to proven products and reputable sellers

- Get the right tools only
- Segment your emails

Chapter 23. When The Warrior Fails

1. Don't take it personally
2. Learn From Your Mistakes
3. Stop Dwelling On Your Failures
4. Model Other Marketers
5. Assess Your Finances
6. Release the Need for Approval from Others
7. Take a Break

Chapter 24. What It All Comes Down To

- Be organized
- Master the fundamentals
- Stick to the basics
- Always have a backup plan
- Stay grounded

Chapter 25. Be A Warrior, Not a Worrier

Chapter 26. The Aim – What it Takes to be a Warrior

Chapter 27. Times You Were Not a Warrior

Chapter 28. The Fire Within

Chapter 29. Finding Your Goal

Chapter 30. Creating Your Own Code of Ethics

Chapter 31. Overcoming Fear

Chapter 32. How to Use 'Fear Setting

Chapter 33. Stoicism and the Warrior Mindset

Chapter 34. Growth Mindset

Chapter 35. Why We Have Become Weak

Chapter 36. How to Get Tough

Chapter 37. Growth Mindset

Chapter 38. Tools for Growth and Resilience

Chapter 39. Correct Breathing

Chapter 40. Cold Showers

Chapter 41. Strength Training and Martial Arts

Chapter 42.Applying Classic Warrior Principles to Business and Life

Chapter 43. Lessons from the Art of War

Chapter 44. Lessons From The Prince

Chapter 45. Conclusion: Taking a Harder Road

Bonus Book - Healthy yourself-

Chapter 46. Introduction

Chapter 47. Know Thy Self

Chapter 48. Know Thy Limits

Chapter 49. Be Honest

Chapter 50. Be Kind

Chapter 51. Be Forgiving

Chapter 52. Be Generous

Chapter 53. Be Yourself

Conclusion

Chapter 1. Introduction

*"A fine line separates a **FIGHTER** from a **WARRIOR**. One is motivated by reason, the other by purpose. One fights to live, while the other lives to fight."*

Hopefully, the quote above inspired you and made you realize that this book that you're reading now is unlike any other. It was written with internet marketers in mind because most of them face certain issues that are very unique.

While most self-help books will congratulate you on taking action and buying these books… that's not going to happen here. All too often, a quote by Lao Tzu is tossed around just to make people feel good… *"A journey of a thousand miles begins with a single step."*

People read this quote and feel very happy when they take the first step. Every New Year's Day, millions of people decide to lose weight and get fit. Their 'single step' involves them paying money and signing up for a gym membership.

This explains why most gyms make most of their money in December and January. The gyms are packed in January with people taking their single step. By March, these same gyms have become ghost towns.

Chapter 2. Why? Why does this happen?

The answer is simple. People focus on the wrong part of the quote. They focus on the words 'single step' instead of the most important word… *"A journey of a thousand miles* **begins** *with a single step."*

'Begins' is the most important word in that quote. Anybody can take that single step and most people do. What happens after that? What happens when you realize that the thousand-mile journey probably requires you to take 10,000 steps?

Will you carry on? Will you take all the steps that you need to?

The hard truth is that most people don't. The journey seems too long. The promise doesn't seem clear anymore. Results aren't coming fast enough… and discouragement sets in.

They quit once the initial sparkle of the first step gets dull. They lose interest and throw in the towel and decide that it's just not worth the effort.

… Until New Year's Day comes around again the following year.

This book will put the fire in your heart to keep going when skies seem dark and the struggles are real. It will give you the strength and guidance to go from the first step to the last one where you attain your goals and dreams.

Thousands of people get on the internet to try and make money. Most quit within the first few months. Out of those who do stay, the majority quit within the first year.

Those who do become successful often realize their goal by sacrificing their health and time with their family. Their business consumes all of their time.

The majority of online marketers are overweight or struggle with health issues. This is not a coincidence. The very nature of online marketing requires one to go through a steep learning curve and it's also very time-consuming.

The initial stages of building a business are hard work before you reach a stage where you can automate your business and earn a passive income. There's just no escaping this fact.

Marketers do their best to do as much as they can at the expense of everything else. There seems to be no other way because of the nature of the internet marketing beast.

This book will show you that being fit and being successful online is not mutually exclusive. You can build a six-figure business and six-pack abs at the same time.

You just need to know the right techniques and the shortcuts so that you do what matters when it matters. This book will teach you simple but highly effective techniques to shed excess pounds.

Want to build muscle? No problem. You'll discover time-saving methods that will get you there as soon as possible.

Trying to get a washboard stomach that will turn heads?

That's covered too.

This book will also cover the emotional and mental issues that so many marketers go through in their online journey. You'll learn to develop mental toughness and resilience to weather the constant challenges that come your way.

There is no fluff and untested theory here. If something can be said in two words, I didn't use three. The methods here work if you work them.

Make a promise to yourself that you'll complete this book and apply what you learn. Knowledge is like paint. It does no good until it's applied.

"Victorious warriors win first and then go to war, while defeated warriors go to war first and then seek to win." – Sun Tzu

What Is Your Why?

Kowing you're why will make all the difference. So what is this 'why' that we're talking about?

It's your reason for doing what you do and make no mistake about this - Your why will always have an emotional reason. You need to dig deep to discover why you want what you want.

If you want to get lean and fit, ask yourself why you want to do it. Be honest. Most people do not want to get in shape for health reasons… That's so boring. Oh no no no! There's always something else.

If men want to get muscular, they probably want to turn women's heads. They want to feel desirable. The same applies to women who want to shed excess pounds. Maybe they want their spouse or partner to look at them in a whole new way.

There's nothing wrong with a little vanity. What matters is that you know why you want what you want.

Some people do it for bragging rights. Others want to prove their naysayers wrong. Then some people just want to achieve something worthy in their life so that they can have the confidence to say that they did at least one thing right.

Even a person who has had a heart attack and recovers will change his eating habits and be more active for an emotional reason. They may fear dying or they want to live so that they can see their kids grow up. **This is the REAL REASON.**

They're not doing it for the sake of being healthy. You must dig deep and self-reflect until you find your underlying reason.

Why do you want to make money online? It's probably not the numbers that excite you.

Saying that you don't have your boss is cool. Being able to brag that nobody controls you anymore and that you live according to your own rules is fun. Being able to buy expensive things without worrying about your finances is beyond fantastic.

These are the emotions that drive you. Your job is to find out what it is… and once you do, **<u>WRITE IT DOWN!</u>**

This is your Warrior Purpose.

If you want, you can even make a video where you record yourself on your mobile phone explaining why your goal is so important to you. It has to be heartfelt. You must be brutally honest with yourself.

Save the video… and keep the paper that you've written you're why on. Always keep them handy.

There will come a point when you're tempted to give up on your goals and dreams. This is inevitable. The universe is challenging you. It may seem all hokey… but you can expect struggles and obstacles to pop-up.

At times like these, you MUST look at the way that you've written down or recorded. Rewrite it if you have to just so you remember and feel what it is you truly wanted.

This will prevent you from throwing in the towel. It will force you to choose between what you want now and what you want most.

If you're tired of starting over, then stop giving up. A warrior

fights to his last. That's his purpose… You're why it is your purpose.

Remember it at all times… and keep refreshing your memory when the initial excitement of taking the first step starts to wane.

Chapter 3. Fighting The Curse of Unrealistic Expectations

This curse has probably killed more dreams than any other reason… but people bring it upon themselves.

Rome wasn't built in a day. This is a very bitter pill to swallow. Success takes time. It takes time to build a business. Losing weight takes time. Building a muscular body takes time.

However, most people are impatient. We live in a world of instant text messaging and microwaves. Everybody wants results fast and they want them now. It just doesn't work that way.

Do not lose faith just because it's taking longer than you thought it would. All things come to he who waits. Keep pushing forward in faith.

Generally, a person can lose about 1 to 2 pounds of fat a week. If you're just starting, you may lose more initially but with time, your results will taper off and you'll probably be at the 1 to 2 pounds per week range.

What if you're 40 pounds overweight? You're looking at a 30 to 40-week stretch to reach your ideal weight. That's about 8 to 9 months!

Most people expect to lose all their excess weight in about 3 weeks. When the results don't come, they lose hope and give up. They never give it enough time.

A warrior takes years to develop his skills. Time is your greatest ally. It doesn't matter what goal you're aiming for. With persistent effort and time, you'll get to your destination.

Keep your expectations realistic. It's good to have a goal that seems out of reach so that you can strive to do your best. Just do not expect to get there overnight.

He who masters patience masters everything else. Avoid this curse at all costs and do not quit just before the results start to come.

Chapter 4. A Warrior Keeps His Promises

When we speak of keeping your promises, it's not just about keeping your promises to other people. You absolutely MUST keep your promises to yourself too.

So few people do this without realizing just how devastating the effects are. If you decide to work out thrice a week, you MUST keep this promise to yourself. If you plan to create content daily for your online business, you must stick to the plan.

There will be times when you just do not feel like it. Times when you're not in the mood. It's during these times that you must take action.

This topic will be addressed in a later chapter. For now, what you need to know is this... When you do not keep your promises to yourself, you lose respect for yourself.

You may give all the excuses you want. As convincing as they may be, deep down on a subconscious level, you'll know that you failed yourself.

Many people hate themselves for not getting to where they want to go in life. It all starts with these little promises that you don't keep.

In the next chapter, we'll look at why you should do what matters when it matters. Respect yourself, your goals and your efforts.

Once you do what you need to do, you'll feel motivated and proud of yourself. This will give you the impetus to keep pushing forward towards your goals.

Chapter 5. Sharpen Your Sword

A warrior's sword is always sharp… and they do not sharpen it during a fight. All preparation and training are done beforehand. They're prepared and ready. They've done what mattered… and this is crucial to success.

Doing what matters is so important that it determines if you'll succeed or just spin your wheels and go nowhere. The world is full of people who are always busy and doing things that are supposed to take them places… but they have no results to show for it.

It always seems like they're not going anywhere but they can't wait to get there. The reason for this is that they mistake activity for work. For example, if you want to lose weight, what matters is that you work out and watch your calories.

Reading a ton of nutrition books, spending hours on YouTube picking up diet tips and joining a gym will not make you lose weight. What matters is the training and what you're eating.

That's all it is… and so many people don't get it. They overwhelm themselves with too much information without taking the right action. The 5 tips below will tell you exactly what you need to do to succeed.

Three tasks a day

Don't make a list of 275 things to get done. That's enough to overwhelm anyone. Start with just 3 tasks… and it must be 3 important tasks. If you're trying to lose weight, the 3 tasks might be a 20-minute stamina workout, intermittent fasting for that day and sleeping early so that you get sufficient rest.

All you need to do are do these 3 tasks. That's it. If you did them over and over, you'll reach your weight loss goal.

Don't live yourself too much work such as studying blood type diets, seeing if the Jupiter is in alignment with Mars so that your chakras will be activated during your yoga session, etc.

All levity aside… focus on just 3 important tasks a day.

Doing just enough to be a little uncomfortable

You must be challenged to grow. If you're trying to build a business online, that may mean writing 2,000 words of content a day. Once you get used to creating this much content with ease, you may wish to push yourself a little and aim for 2,500 words.

You want to be making gradual progress. Over time, you'll be amazed at how it all adds up.

The same applies to your fitness. If you can only run for 10 minutes on the treadmill, that's ok. With each workout, try and increase the duration by 20 seconds.

The difference will be a little uncomfortable but it won't be so bad that it scares you. Make measurable progress in a reasonable time.

Do the most difficult task first

It's human nature to do everything else but the most difficult task. You might decide to rearrange your desk or sort out your folders on your computer when what you need to do is analyze the statistics in your advertising account.

The mind tries to escape the difficult tasks. Your job is to do them first. Forget everything else and just do the most difficult task at once. Focus on that. Once that is complete, it'll be a weight off your chest and the rest of the lesser tasks will be completed with ease.

Activity and work are two different things

As mentioned earlier, you must know the difference. Streamline your life so that you're only doing what matters. Do not do unnecessary stuff. Eliminate all the trivial jobs that don't contribute to your progress.

Then you'll have more time to do what matters.

Know when to take a break

Music is the space between the notes. Take short breaks every time you feel a little tired. This will keep you focused and more energetic to complete the important stuff.

That's all there is to it.

"Don't tell me how busy you are. Show me what you've gotten done. Words don't matter. Results do." – Larry Winget

Chapter 6. The Importance of Focus

Bruce Lee once said, *"Concentration is the root of all the higher abilities in man."*

To succeed in life, you must have the ability to focus and concentrate. Focused hard work is the key to success. The best way to focus is to remove all distractions.

But the focus is slightly more than just removing distractions. In our day and age, multitasking is said to be a useful skill.

In truth, you should avoid multitasking. It distracts you and over time you'll lose the ability to stay focused on any one thing for long.

You'll never see a warrior engaged in a sword fight and taking quick peeps at his Facebook wall to see what's up. 100% focus on the fight in front of you.

Aim to do just one task at a time and give it your best. You must know how long you can last while concentrating. Some people can focus for an entire hour without getting exhausted… while others may get tired after just 20 minutes.

Do what suits you best. If you need a mental break, take it. Spend 5 minutes resting and come back and focus on your task again. Over time, your 'stamina' will increase.

It's crucial to develop focus if you want to be mentally strong. The successful warrior is the average man with a laser-like focus.

Chapter 7. Battling The Fear "Demons"

Everyone has fears and this is inevitable. It is part and parcel of life. However, what separates the winners from the masses who fail is the ability to acknowledge one's fears and push through them.

While conquering one's deepest and darkest fears is not easy, it is definitely worth the effort. As an online marketer, there will be times when the skies seem gloomy and you wonder if it will all work out.

Financial insecurities, temporary setbacks and the usual challenges that life throws at you can be daunting. The majority of beginners will throw in the towel and quit the moment the going gets tough.

They falsely believe that they don't have what it takes to succeed or the journey is just too tough for them. They fear the 'hard

yards' and the travails that must be endured for one to see success. They quit out of fear.

But you're different because you know better. When it comes to fear, you only have 2 choices.

1. **F**orget **E**verything **A**nd **R**un **Or**
2. **F**ace **E**verything **A**nd **R**ise

The choice is quite obvious. While the first one will be easy, it will leave you stranded in the muck and mire of mediocrity. Your dreams and goals will die from strangulation by fear.

Choose the second option and you'll push past your fear with grim determination. When you come out on the other side, you'll be emotionally stronger, mentally tougher and you'll taste the fruits of success.

There is no other way. You only have 2 options. Choose the second one. Everything you want is on the other side of fear.

In this guide, we'll look at 5 of the most common fears that plague most online marketers and how you can calm your beating heart.

Fear of the Unknown

This is probably one of the biggest fears that entrepreneurs face. When you're starting your own business, while you may have done your homework and prepared the best you can, there will ALWAYS be a certain degree of uncertainty. That's just the way it is.

You must always remember that you can't discover new lands if you're afraid to lose sight of the shore. You have to push through and go with your heart, even if it's beating uncontrollably fast.

Sometime in 1999, there was a movie called "3 Kings". In one scene in the movie, a young soldier who was feeling afraid would approach Sergeant Major Archie Gates (George Clooney) with a question and he'd reply... *"The way these works is... You do the thing you're scared sh*tless of and you get the courage after you do it. Not before you do it."*

This is very true and it applies across the board. If you're worried that you may not have the skills to create an online business, go ahead and do it anyway. Then learn as you go along.

You must have the faith to take the first step even when you can't see the whole staircase. The best way to put an end to your fear of the unknown is to have faith.

You must believe in yourself and what you're trying to achieve. There are thousands of people who come online in droves hoping to make quick and easy money. Most of them fail and quit.

The road to online success is paved with the corpses of the many who have tried and quit. They quit because they didn't believe in themselves and they let fear take over.

Like John Stewart Mill said, *"One person with a belief is equal to a force of ninety-nine who only have an interest."*

The next time you have doubts and fears, ask yourself why you're feeling them. Maybe you've been making a stable income online but you're worried about quitting your day job because of the security it provides.

By asking yourself why you have this fear, you'll understand that what you fear is that you might have no money in case your online business dries up.

Now you'll be able to make plans such as saving up enough money that will last you six months in case of any unexpected setbacks. This is a plan of action.

If you do not analyze your fears and all you do is let them control you and hold you back, your life will become stagnant and in almost all cases, there will be retrogression.

The only way to progress is to keep moving forward whether or not you have fears.

The Fear of Failure

This is another major fear that paralyzes so many marketers from taking action on their goals and dreams. The fear of failure has stopped more people in their tracks than any other fear.

Usually, this fear is disguised in many different ways. If you worry that all your efforts will go to waste when your online efforts earn you no money, that's a fear of failure. Most people say that they just 'don't want to waste their time on something that won't work.'

The hard truth is that you'll never know unless you try. It may take you 3 years to build an online business that's making you six figures a year. But guess what? If you don't try because you're scared that you'll fail, the time is going to pass anyway.

The 3 years will go by and chances are your life will probably be the same. Whereas if you had moved forward with your goals, you just might be in the six-figure income category.

A lot of people fear failure because it will make them look foolish in front of their friends and family. They do not want to endure criticism or sneers from their peers.

This fear is unnecessary. What others think of you should be the least of your concerns. You may notice that when you try to better yourself and do things that others don't do, your friends and family will probably be your hardest critics and they'll call it 'concern' or 'tough love.'

The truth of the matter is that you making progress and achieving your goals shines a spotlight on their failures. It makes them feel threatened and the only way for them to feel better is to drag you down to their level so that the status quo can be maintained.

This is life and by understanding that what others think of you is none of your business, this fear of looking foolish will disappear all on its own.

Lao Tzu once said, *"Care about what other people think and you will always be their prisoner."*

The best way to deal with the fear of failure is to ask yourself what could go wrong. Now plan out what countermeasures you can take to prevent your endeavors from failing.

Spend time visualizing yourself pushing past obstacles and succeeding. Repeat this visualization process daily... and even a

couple of times a day. This will give you faith and belief in yourself to keep going forward.

The Fear That You Are Not Good Enough

This fear arises when one has failed several times throughout life. Many people do not do well academically while in school because they had no natural affinity to the subjects they were learning.

The girl who was gifted at art probably failed at math and science and couldn't go further than high school. This failure may make her feel like she can't succeed at anything in life... even though she has all the potential to be a successful artist.

The very wise Albert Einstein once said, *"Everyone is a genius. But if you judge a fish by its ability to climb a tree, it will live its whole life believing that it is stupid."*

The point of that statement is that one should not judge themselves based on how they performed in school or previous jobs.

There are countless stories of people who failed many times and finally succeeded beyond their wildest dreams once they found their true calling. Never give up on yourself. Fortune favors the bold.

Usually, when you're trying to build an online business, there will be a learning curve that you'll have to go through. This is inevitable.

You will make mistakes. You will buy products that are rubbish… And you will waste time and money. This too is normal and can't be avoided. However, if you quit while at this stage because you feel like you're not good enough, you'll NEVER get better.

You only get better as you keep learning and progressing. Many beginners look at expert marketers and feel intimidated. They believe that the other guys are smarter, richer and better than them.

Do not compare yourself with others. This is a huge mistake and will always leave you feeling discontented. You may be comparing your beginning with someone else's finish. It's not fair to you and you'll be doing yourself a disservice. All you need to do is focus on being the best that you can be.

Here's the truth. Everybody started as a beginner. You do not become successful overnight. There is a journey that you have to go through and go through it you must.

Fearing that you'll never amount to much will mean that you have given up before you even started. You must have confidence.

Chalk up every little failure that you encounter along the way as a learning experience. You can't extrapolate from incomplete data. The more you learn, the better you'll get.

The more mistakes you make the better. Failure is not the opposite of success. It is a part of success. You are good enough. You've always been. You just need to believe it.

The Fear That You're Late or Too Old

This is another big one. You may have heard terms like 'Article marketing is dead… or 'The good ol' days are over'… 'You're too old to start a business'… But are these statements even true?

Of course not. While some methods may come and go, building a business online is here to stay and every single day people are reaching their income goals. It's never too late to start and now is as good a time as any.

You're also never too old to set new goals or dream new dreams. Stan Lee created his first hit comic close to his 39th birthday.

Henry Ford was 45 when he created the Model T car. Ray Croc only started MacDonald's at the age of 52 and Colonel Sanders was 62 when he franchised KFC.

As you can see, people have succeeded in life at all ages. You're never too old. So cast this fear aside and pursue your dreams today.

"The best time to plant a tree was 20 years ago. The second best time is now." – Chinese proverb,

Limiting Beliefs

Just when you were expecting another fear, you've been hit with 'limiting beliefs'... It may be surprising but it's true. Many people have been held back from success because of their own beliefs.

There is an emotional disconnect within them. The reason for this is that while growing up, we formed our beliefs based on what we saw, what we heard and what we were told.

One good example will be overweight people who feel like they're 'destined' to be fat. Their parents, siblings, relatives, and everyone close to them are overweight so they buy into the story that they are naturally predisposed to obesity.

While to a certain extent it could be true because some people have a naturally slower metabolism, the truth of the matter is that food choice, eating habits, attitudes towards food, etc. are often passed down from parents to the kids.

Because of this, all they ever knew about food and eating is what they saw and heard. If they decided to eat clean, exercise more and watch their calories, they'd definitely lose all the excess pounds and probably end up being the leanest person in their family.

But getting to this stage requires one to overcome their limited thinking and believe that they are worthy of success.

The same applies to people who grew up in poor families where the parents made it look like money was hard to come by or that rich people were evil and greedy… while poor people were generous and kind.

With beliefs like these, their subconscious mind will not allow them to build wealth because they wouldn't want to be evil and greedy, would they?

Overcoming your limited self-beliefs is a Herculean task but it can be done. You will need to be proactive and be alert to the way you think and correct yourself.

Once you realize that your only limit is you, your life will change and you'll conquer this obstacle. You are worthy of success.

By now you'll realize that fear is **false** **e**vidence **a**ppearing **r**eal. The best way to conquer fear is through action. Analyzing why you feel the way you feel is helpful… but nothing beats action when it comes to dispelling fear. Do what you fear most and the fear will vanish.

Never let your fear decide your future. Make a good plan, have contingencies in place and work your plan till you succeed. Even during the darkest hours when everything around you may feel like it's all about to collapse and all your fears are telling you that you're about to fail… dig your heels in and keep pushing forward.It's always darkest before the dawn. Keep going.

Chapter 8. Climb The Staircase That You Can't See

There's a saying that goes, "Faith is seeing light with your heart when all your eyes see is darkness." This is very true and when you're trying to build a business, facing problems, hiccups, disappointments and other 'turbulence' are unavoidable.

Most people quit and run the other way once things seem to not be working out. They lose hope and throw in the towel. They do not believe success is within their reach and they assume that it's not possible.

Why?

Because they've lost faith. There is no other explanation for this. A loss of faith in one's self is the number one reason most peoplequit on themselves. The promise isn't clear to them so they're not willing to pay the price.

However, the people who are single-minded and cannot see anything but themselves reaching their goal will often weather the storms and obstacles to get to where they want to go… and they almost always reach their goals.

Faith is of paramount importance. **It means taking the first step even when you don't see the whole staircase.**

The 4 tips listed below will help you shore up your faith when doubts come knocking on your door.

Visualize your success

Some people call it the law of attraction. Others call it 'The Secret'. Whatever you want to call it… what matters is that you do it.

Close your eyes and see yourself reaching your goals and attaining your heartfelt desires. Believe that you'll get them and live with an attitude that your success is just around the corner.

This will keep you feeling upbeat and the constant repetition will give you focus and make you remember why you're doing what you do.

Prayer is powerful

While this may not apply to atheists, if you do believe in God, there is immeasurable power in prayer. You will be placing your faith and hopes in a higher power and this will lift some of the burdens weighing on you.

It doesn't matter what religion you follow. It's the action of having hope and faith that your God will help you which is what truly matters.

Read autobiographies of successful people

ea to read the autobiographies of successful

people. You'll be able to see how many failures they encountered and how they kept going. You'll be able to identify with them and realize that the path to success is not a smooth one.

If they could achieve success, so can you. This will bolster your faith in yourself… and your faith will be bigger than your fears of failure.

Motivate yourself regularly

The famous motivational speaker, Zig Ziglar once said, "People often say that motivation doesn't last. Well, neither does bathing

- that's why we recommend it daily."

He's right. It's easy to lose motivation and faith over time. Once the initial excitement of starting on a new goal starts to get dull, most people quit. By constantly motivating yourself, you'll keep going.

Read books or listen to motivational speakers. While some people will scoff and say that it's all 'feel good' stuff… just know that it will you if you give it a chance.

Building a successful business is not easy. If it was, everybody will do it. So, have faith in yourself and know that if you stay the course, success is inevitable. To succeed, you must first believe that you can… and then you will.

Chapter 9. A Tiger Doesn't Lose Sleep Over The Opinions Of Sheep.

Call them what you want… naysayers, haters, wet blankets, etc. but the sad truth is that more dreams have been killed by negative people than anything else.

The truly successful people in life never gave two hoots what other people thought of them. They just carried on focusing on their goals and strived till they made their dreams come true.

When you have a dream or a desire in life, you must follow your heart. You only have one life to live and you do not want to reach old age where you have no energy and time left to make your dreams come true.

Having regrets when you're old is sad. Your past desires and dreams will return to haunt you and you'll realize that you could have done so much more or been so much more… but you let yourself get discouraged by those who didn't let you be you.

By now, it will be too late and you'll realize that none of what other people said mattered… and you should have followed your heart. This is a sad scenario but it plays out daily in thousands of people's lives.

You do not want to end up like them. These six tips below will help you to handle naysayers and not let them get you down.

Look at your why

Only you will know why your dreams are so important to you. Maybe you have a love for art and a natural inclination towards it but your parents want you to be a doctor.

Maybe you have a desire to start your own business but your wife is skeptical and thinks that your day job provides more security.

What are you going to do?

If you know why you're doing what you do, you'll push ahead despite what others tell you. The promise will be clear to you and you'll go against your critics.

Remember the bamboo tree

There is a story about Chinese bamboo. Once you plant the seed, you'll need to water the soil for 5 years. During these 5 years, nothing will happen. However, in the 5th year, a shoot will sprout out from the ground.

Once that happens, over the next 6 weeks, it will grow over 80 feet tall. That's amazing.

The same applies to your goals. It may seem like ages to get there and of course, people will be hinting at you that you might as well quit. Yet, if you persist, once you take off, your success will be massive.

Get motivated

When you're feeling down because people have poured water on your dreams or told you that you're destined to fail, do listen to motivational videos or read motivational books to pick yourself up.

Know that it's all turbulence

When a plane takes off from the ground, many times it will face turbulence as it rises above the weather to reach cruising altitude. In the same vein, the beginning stages of getting to your goal will be tough, but once you get there, it will most often be smooth sailing.

Success turns naysayers into supporters

It's a fact that the same people who laughed at you and mocked you will become your supporters once you make it.

They'll ask you for tips and advice to help themselves achieve success just like you. If you build a successful business, people who doubted you will even ask you for a job. That's just the way the world is.

Understand the psychology behind it

Lastly, you need to understand that when you pursue your dreams, you are like a threat to others. Your determination to follow your

path and live life according to your own rules shines a spotlight on the failures of those around you.

It forces people to realize that they quit on themselves or did not do enough. The only way that they can feel better is to pull you down so that you can be a failure just like them.

They may make you feel like they're doing it out of concern. But the truth of the matter is that they're afraid you'll succeed…

because if you do, it'll mean that they could have followed their dreams and succeeded too.

Always follow your warrior's heart and don't allow the negativity from others to dull your sparkle or your desires.

Chapter 10. Weight Loss Is Simpler Than You Think

It is extremely common to gain weight when you devote all your time to work at the expense of everything else. Anyone who has tried to build a business online will realize just how time-consuming it is.

It is quite a journey to go from the newbie stage to the level where you earn profits while you sleep… Or live the laptop lifestyle where you make thousands of dollars in twenty minutes while you lie back on some sun-kissed tropical beach.

Most marketers are at the stage where they're struggling to make it work. They let their health slide. They barely exercise. They develop poor eating habits, drink too much coffee and sleep at odd hours.

While it may not seem like a big deal, the pounds will slowly start creeping in. You'll start gaining weight, your metabolism will

drop, your energy levels will dip and while your income levels may climb, you will be inviting potential health problems into your life.

This is a very real scenario and many marketers struggle to get their weight under control once they realize how far they've let themselves go. They then put themselves through ridiculous diets or decide to go crazy at the gym.

It all feels torturous and they often quit and resign themselves to being fat. It doesn't have to be that way. You can be lean and fit while building your online business.

Now you're going to learn 8 simple weight loss tips that will keep you from gaining unnecessary weight. The most important thing to know is that **80 percent of your results come from your diet**.

Just by paying attention to what you eat, you'll be able to prevent weight gain. After all, you only want to see your income go up and not the numbers on the weighing scale.

In the fitness industry, there is a saying, *"Abs are made in the kitchen, not the gym."*

It just means that your diet is much more important than exercise when it comes to staying lean. You absolutely can't out-exercise a bad diet.

Before going further, we need to talk about something very important… **Your Attitude.**

Most people are impatient and want results fast. Your goal should be different. You should be in this for the long haul. Since you're trying to build a business online, in most cases, you'll be crunched for time.

You just can't afford to spend hours at the gym. Some of the top marketers are so busy that they can only spare time to exercise thrice a week.

So the goal here will be to make gradual improvements over time. As long as you're taking the right steps, you will see results gradually. Instead of struggling with a lemonade diet for 3 weeks, you could follow simpler steps that will get you to the same results in about 5 weeks.

Time is your greatest ally and since your focus is on marketing instead of looking like a Greek God, there is no real rush here. The slow approach is far more effective in the long run than the short bursts that most people try to do. You're creating healthy habits that will last you a lifetime. Now let's look at what you need to do.

Cut the carbs

This single action alone will make a HUGE difference in your weight. Studies have shown that a diet that restricts carb intake is far more effective than a diet that restricts calorie intake.

First, you'll need to know what your daily calorie numbers should be. You can find that out here: http://www.freedieting.com/tools/calorie_calculator.htm

Now that you know what your calorie deficit should be, your focus should be to get most of your calories from protein and fats. Do not worry about consuming fats. You need to eat fat to lose fat. It may sound contradictory but it's true.

Once your body realizes that it's getting a regular intake of fat, it will be more willing to burn its fat stores since there is no real need to retain fat unnecessarily.

As long as you're at a caloric deficit, you will lose weight. Just ensure that you're consuming 50 grams or less of carbs. This is crucial.

The goal here is to go for 3 to 5 days with very low carb intake and then follow up with a day where you consume carbs as normal. This is known as a re-feed day or 'cheat' day.

When you consume carbs again after a few days of minimal carbohydrate intake, you'll replenish your body's glycogen stores and give your metabolic rate a boost. Your body will not go into 'starvation mode' where it stubbornly clings on to its fat stores.

It will start burning more fat now that you have elevated your metabolism again. This method of eating is known as 'carb cycling' and it's used by fitness models all over the world to stay lean and ripped.

As an online marketer, this is not a huge change to make. You'll just be eating a little less daily because of the 500 calorie deficit required… and you'll be consuming fewer carbs.

It will be slightly difficult initially… but it's not as difficult as switching to a paleo diet or an Atkins diet that takes things to an extreme. All you need to do is switch some of your carb foods to protein foods.

Make gradual changes and you'll find it more bearable. Inch by inch, life is a cinch. Yard by yard, life is hard.

Do note: Of all the 8 tips listed in this book, this is the most important one as far as losing weight goes. If you just get this tip right, you will lose weight. *Your diet is of paramount importance to weight loss.*

Intermittent fasting

The second tip to weight loss is intermittent fasting, also known as IF. This is a method of eating that doesn't require you to do much other than eat at different times.

Once you have switched to a carb cycling method of eating, you will need to combine it with intermittent fasting to accelerate your weight loss.

In simple words, intermittent fasting has two windows. There is the eating window and the fasting window. In most cases, the eating window is 8 hours and the fasting window is 16 hours… and in total, that's a day.

All your calories will need to be consumed during the eating window. For example, if you start your day having breakfast at 8 am, your last meal for the day should end at 4 pm. That's your 8-hour eating window. You can't eat anything after that but you can drink water.

By doing this, your body will have much more time to tap into its fat stores for fuel since it has not much food left to burn.

Intermittent fasting, when combined with carb cycling, is extremely potent at shedding the excess pounds.

You'll need to decide for yourself when you want to start your eating window. Some people need breakfast when they wake… while others prefer sleeping with a full stomach.

There are no hard and fast rules here. As long as you eat within the window, it doesn't matter when you start your first meal. An interesting point to note is that the smaller your eating window, the more fat you'll lose.

For example, if your eating window is 5 or 6 hours, it will be more effective than an 8-hour window because your body has more time to tap into its fat stores for fuel.

Another point to note is that you will not be starving yourself. After all, you are getting all the calories you need for the day. You're just getting them in a shorter time frame.

Give intermittent fasting a try and you'll see how effective it is. Initially, it will be tough for the first week or so, but once you get the hang of it, your body will adapt and the fat will melt off.

Get enough sleep

You absolutely must get enough sleep every day. It is very common for marketers to burn the candle at both ends and sacrifice sleep to get more work done. Once in awhile is fine… but this should not become a habit.

A lack of sleep indirectly leads to weight gain. You become more stressed out and your body releases the stress hormone cortisol. You'll end up feeling hungry or binge eating for no real reason.

Get 7 to 8 hours of sleep. Some people may be able to function well with just 5 or 6 hours. It all depends on the individual. Just know that if you're struggling to wake up, you need more sleep.

Fasted cardio

This is another simple but very effective tip. When you wake up in the morning, your body is in a fasted state and your glycogen levels are low.

This is the best time to do some light exercise. Just 20 to 30 minutes will do. It could be walking, cycling, swimming or any cardio activity.

The key point to note is that it has to be at an intensity that allows you to break a light sweat but not one where you're gasping for breath.

For example, if you're doing a brisk walk, you should be able to comfortably hold a conversation. That's a good place to maintain. What matters is that you do this exercise on an empty stomach.

Your body will tap into its fat stores for fuel because there is no food in the belly for it to use. You'll be burning fat immediately.

So, if you can spare 20 to 30 minutes in the morning, go for a brisk walk and over time, you'll have lost more weight and also feel more energetic.

Shorter but higher intensity workouts

As was mentioned earlier, marketers generally do not have much time. Those with day jobs and family commitments have even less time. This is NOT a problem when it comes to exercise.

All too often we hear people say that they *just don't have time to exercise.'*

While this may be true to a certain extent, there is absolutely no doubt that anyone can spare 10 minutes to exercise. Here's the catch. The workout has to be at maximum intensity.

You could work out for just 15 minutes thrice a week and be very fit. The goal here is to train at maximum intensity. You want to aim for full-body workouts or training methods that are exhausting.

One good example would be sprints. A 10-minute interval workout with you sprinting for 1 minute followed by a rest of 1 minute repeated over and over till the time is up will be far more effective than a 45-minute slow jog.

You'd be surprised to know that even 4 minutes can put you in fat-burning mode. Do check out what the Tabata Protocol is and try to do it if you're interested.

A 15-minute workout is 1 percent of your day. Anyone can spare time for it.

Eat Foods That Burn Fat

Some foods have been shown to burn more fat than others due to the thermogenic effect of food and even the properties of the

food. Below you'll find a list. Do include these foods in your diet.

- Avocado

- Organic Apple Cider Vinegar

- Green Tea

- Broccoli

- Healthy Eggs

- Flax Seeds

- Hot Peppers

- Chicken Breast

- Greek Yogurt
- Salmon

- Onions

- Blueberries

- Cinnamon

- Spinach

- Olive Oil

Drink Lots of Water

This is a very simple tip. The body needs water to stay hydrated and metabolize fat. Set a timer on your watch to go off once every hour. Drink a glass of water when the timer goes off. Easy and consistent.

Drink a glass of water before every meal. It will make you feel fuller and you will be less inclined to eat more than you need to. This action can help to curb your appetite.

Have a Food Journal

Write down everything you eat and drink for the day. Now you

have a written record that will show you where you're slipping up. All you need to do is replace unhealthy food choices with healthier ones.

The goal here is to make small positive changes that are easy to comply with. Go from 3 sodas a day to 2 a day. Don't suddenly cut out all 3 and switch to unsweetened green tea. Compliance will be a nightmare and you'll probably end up drinking 5 sodas a day. Go slow and make gradual progress.

If you follow these 8 tips, your weight loss progress will skyrocket. Since you lack time, what you do must count. These are some of the most effective weight loss tips out there.

They do not require massive changes or too much time. Any online marketer can follow these tips without disrupting their life.

So, implement these tips and you'll look better, feel better and be proud of your body.

Chapter 11. From Ideal Weight To A Six Pack

In this chapter, you'll be given the exact information to get a six-pack. It's easier than most people realize.

Ideally, you should have used the tips from the previous chapter to reach your ideal weight. You can find out your ideal weight here - http://www.calculator.net/ideal-weight-calculator.html

You have no business struggling with sit-ups and talking about a six-pack if you're 30 pounds overweight. Getting a six-pack requires you to first be at your ideal weight.

From there, you'll lower your bodyfat percentage till you reach the single digits. In bodybuilding, they call it being vascular. Men will see their six-packs once they're at 6 to 9 percent body fat.

Women will see it when they're at 16 to 19 percent body fat.

So how do you get there?

Chapter 12. Calories

As an online marketer, you probably are too busy to slave away at the gym for hours. The truth is that you do not need to. All you need to do is follow the tips that you learned earlier to keep your body in fat-burning mode.

You must monitor your calories very closely. You can see the calculation below.

To see a 2-pack – (Bodyweight in pounds X 13) calories To see a 4-pack – Bodyweight in pounds X 12) calories To see a 6-pack – (Bodyweight in pounds X 11) calories

You're taking your weight in pounds and multiplying it by the numbers shown. So, if you weigh 160 pounds, you should be consuming no more than 2,080 calories a day till you see

your 2-pack, which is your top 2 abs muscles. Then drop your calorie intake to your current weight multiplied by 11.

<u>Make sure you go progressively</u>. Do not start with your bodyweight and multiply it by 10 just so you can get your six-pack faster. You'll just end up hitting a plateau and see no progress.

Chapter 13. Training

Now that the calorie part is taken care of, you'll need to make sure that most of your workouts are at maximum intensity.

You must be gasping and struggling as you workout. Nothing but you're very best! This will create a situation known as EPOC – excess post-exercise oxygen consumption.

Once you reach this stage, your body will be in fat-burning mode for 10 to 14 hours after your workout. The fat will just melt off.

Do full-body workouts that include exercises such as:

- Deadlifts

- Pull-ups

- Lunges

- Squats

- Snatches

- Mountain climbers

- Burpees

- Bench presses

- Hanging leg raises

These are compound movements. It's a great idea to use weights. Unlike earlier when you were just trying to shed the excess pounds, now you're trying to burn the last and most stubborn layer of fat.

You only need to do about 20 to 30 minutes. There's no need for 45-minute or 60-minute workouts. Short fast workouts are what matters.

Always lift as much weight as you can fast and with good form. If your form is wobbly or you're slow, the weights are too heavy.

Use lighter weights that are manageable but still challenging.

Chapter 14. Diet

By now, you should have instilled some discipline in your eating.

Here's an important point to note. When trying to shed excess fat, as long as you're at a caloric deficit, you'll lose weight.

What you eat while important, is not didn't have much of an impact. You could sneak in junk food now and then and still lose weight as long as you consume fewer calories than you expend.

To get six-pack abs, **your diet will be a lot less forgiving**. Not all calories are made equal. You'll need to clean up your diet as much as you can.

A bar of chocolate that has 200 calories is a lot more detrimental than a slice of steak that is also 200 calories. While the numbers are the same, the chocolate will cause your blood sugar levels to spike.

Your body will release insulin which will lead to weight gain... or at the very least, it will be much more difficult to burn off the last stubborn layer of fat on your lower abdomen that doesn't want to leave.

Avoid processed foods and dairy as much as you can. Stick to single-ingredient foods such as broccoli, chicken breast, etc. Your body can only take in so many calories and every calorie has to count.

You should consume most of your calories in protein and fat. This is known as a ketogenic diet. You must eat fat to lose fat. Add extra virgin olive oil or cold-pressed coconut oil during your food preparation.

As long as there are sufficient fat and proteins in your diet and about 50 grams of carbs daily, you'll reach your six-pack within 4 to 7 weeks. To speed things up, incorporate intermittent fasting into your program and have a 5 or 6-hour eating window.

Another thing to be aware of is that for each gram of carbohydrates that you consume, your body will hold on to 3 grams of water. So, if on one particular day you consume more carbs, your weight will rise the next day due to water retention.

You can solve this problem by drinking a lot more water on that day to flush out the excess water. The same applies if you eat foods high in salt. It seems contradictory that one should drink more water to reduce water retention. But that's how it is.

That's all there is to it. You do not need to spend countless hours at the gym or do thousands of sit-ups. **3 to 4 short but intense workouts a week is more than enough to get your six-pack**.

Chapter 15. Building Muscle and Gaining Mass

Generally, it's best to get a six-pack first before you attempt to bulk up. While getting a six-pack requires you to be at a caloric deficit, building muscle and gaining mass requires you to be at a caloric surplus.

As an online marketer, you probably don't have the time to dedicate to working out one body part a day. So, you need a split.

Once again, the goal is 3 workouts a week – about 30 to 40 minutes each. You do not need to go above that. You can if you want to, but it isn't necessary. Let's look at an example of a 3-day split.

Monday – Legs/calves Tuesday – Rest

Wednesday – Chest/shoulders/triceps Thursday – Rest

Friday – Back/biceps/forearms

That's an excellent split and it's manageable. There are so many different exercises to target each muscle. It would be best to do research and vary your workouts.

Generally, these are the most crucial and effective exercises. If all you did were these exercises, you would be fine.

- Legs – Barbell squats, calf raises, dumbbell lunges

- Biceps – Hammer curls, EZ bar curls, incline hammer curls, bicep curls
- Triceps – Skullcrushers, push-ups, triceps pushdowns, close grip bench press
- Chest – Barbell bench press, incline bench press, dips, incline dumbbell flyes
- Forearms – Seated wrist curls, wrist rollers, farmer's walk
- Back – Deadlifts, wide grip pull-ups, single-arm dumbbell rows, snatches
- Shoulders – Front/side/rear lateral raises, Arnold press.

Chapter 16. How many reps and sets?

All you need to do is 8 to 12 reps per exercise for 4 to 5 sets. Lift as much weight as you can to barely make these reps. You want to be challenging yourself.

You do not always need to train to failure. Training to failure is a strategy that should be employed once every 3 workouts.

Training to failure means that on your last set of each exercise, you keep doing reps until a point where you just can't do another one more rep. Your muscles will be burning and all good form goes out the window.

This will cause micro-tears in your muscles and when the scars heal, there'll be more muscle tissue. **Do note that you should take a 1-week break every 8 weeks.** Do not exercise during this entire week. Let your body heal.

As far as nutrition goes, **you should multiply your body weight in pounds by 20 to know how many calories you should be consuming**. It's a good idea to get most of your calories from clean, nutritious food.

But sometimes, that can be difficult and tiring. It's perfectly fine to eat some junk food to meet the calorie count. This is known as a 'dirty bulk.'

Will you gain weight? Yes... but you'll also gain muscle. Do not worry too much about gaining fat. You can do a 'cut' later where you burn off the excess fat. You already know what you need to know to lose weight.

Ideally, you should bulk for 2 or 3 months and then do a cut where you go on a caloric deficit and burn fat. Keep your diet clean during this period and do not do more than 2 or 3 high-intensity workouts a week... and keep them within the 15 to 20-minute duration.

You just want to boost your metabolism so that your body goes into the fat-burning mode. As long as your diet is on point and clean, you'll shed the excess pounds but now you'll have more muscle mass.

Do not let yourself get too overweight before you decide to do a cut. Monitor your weight closely.

Some men find it extremely hard to bulk up. These are usually ectomorph body types with a high metabolic rate. If you face this issue, you'll need to aim for a 1,000 to 2,000 calorie a day surplus over and above the number you calculated earlier.

You'll feel sick of eating but it's a necessary evil. All cardio training should be limited to just walking for about 20 minutes twice or thrice a week.

Never workout more than thrice a week. You can even workout twice a week and it may yield better results. Less is more... and while it seems countcrintuitive, this is what an ectomorph needs to do.

As with all things, consistency is the most important thing. Since it's just 3 times a week and the workouts are about 30 minutes long, it's manageable.

Chapter 17. How much muscle can I hope to gain?

According to Lyle Macdonald's Natural Lean Muscle Mass Gain

Model... this is what you can expect. It's a pretty accurate guide.

Year 1 - 20-25 pounds (2 pounds per month)

Year 2 - 10-12 pounds (1 pound per month)

Year 3 - 5-6 pounds (.5 pound per month)

Year 4 and on - 2-3 pounds (not worth calculating).

As you can see, it takes time to build muscle and as the years pass, it gets more difficult. So, tailor your expectations accordingly and stay the course. Consistency is the key. If you can't be consistent, you can't be anything.

Before you start with weights...

Here's something that most gym trainers will not tell you. Before you even sign up for a gym membership or start training with weights, make sure you put yourself through about 8 weeks of solid bodyweight training.

Some so many beginners do bicep curls and hammer

curls at the gym... but they can't do a single pull-up. Ask them to do 30 push-ups at a go and they struggle.

Build a strong foundation by doing as much bodyweight training as you can. Your muscles and ligaments will get used to

resistance training... and you'll be amazed to discover that even guys who are built like a house, struggle with bodyweight exercises such as the V-sit, muscle up, human flag, archer push-ups, etc.

Go on YouTube and find as many different bodyweight exercises that you can and do them till you are good at them and much stronger. Now you have a solid foundation in resistance training... you're ready for weights at the gym.

Chapter 18. Don't neglect your posture and flexibility

Make sure you stretch often and always maintain good posture. As a marketer who spends hours in front of the computer, do make sure you stretch your neck, shoulders, back and do head rotations.

This will prevent chronic issues from arising. Get up off your seat for 5 minutes every hour and do some stretches. This is very important. If you can, practice yoga and Pilates. This will be very beneficial in the long run.

Resistance training will make your muscles tighter. There will be a loss of range of motion. To solve this problem, do some light stretching daily.

A Warrior Watches His Money

As far as getting lean, fit and muscular go, you already know all you need to know. Now you need to know an important truth – How to manage your money and when is the right time to quit your day job.

The majority of people who try and make money online do so because they wish to quit their day job. They hate the commute, the lack of freedom, their unreasonable bosses, their backstabbing colleagues… and the list of woes goes on.

It all seems so nice to be able to work from home. No commute. Freedom to do what you want, when you want and nobody to boss you around. It's fantastic.

The big question is… **When do you quit your day job?**

Many marketers make a huge mistake here and quit their day job way too early. They decide to give internet marketing their full attention and it's either make it or break it. They believe that they're bold and taking the right action.

Nothing could be further from the truth.

Make it or break it? Almost all the time, these marketers break it and fail on an epic level. They become broke, in debt and finally end up getting another job. They then feel bitter and give up on internet marketing.

What they don't realize is that they could have made it if they only knew when to quit their day job… and this is what they should have looked out for.

What's your number?

Your number refers to the amount of money you need to survive every month. A good estimate will be your current salary multiplied by 1.5.

If you are earning this amount consistently every month for 5 to 6 months, you are ready to quit. The reason it is 1.5 and not one is because your income can fluctuate wildly at times and the extra 0.5 is just to take up the slack should you earn less any single month.

You do not want to be in a situation where you can't afford your rent just because your website was down for a week due to some issues.

Money is oxygen to your business

You need money to build an online business. Your day job will provide you that money to invest in your business. As long as your online business is incapable of sustaining itself from its earnings, you are not ready to quit your day job yet.

Use a portion of your monthly salary to invest in your business. Work at your day job while you build your fortune. Once you are raking in dollars, you can toss in your resignation.

Can you do both effectively?

This is an interesting question. Many people do not hate their day job. They just hate their salary. If you have an online income that's making you an extra two thousand a month, life at your job may suddenly seem much better since you have more cash now.

If that's the case and you like your day job and colleagues, there's no need to quit. You can automate and outsource your business so that you can have both a job and an online income.

Your six-month nest egg

Before quitting your day job, make sure you have at least 6 months of your current salary saved up. This will be a buffer if there is an emergency or if your business suddenly fails.

You'll have time to fix the problems or at the very least, find a new job.

Insurance and medical benefits

Most jobs have some form of insurance or medical benefits such as dental coverage, etc. Make sure you're earning enough online to cover all these costs. There's more than just a monthly wage that you should be looking at.

Is your spouse working?

Yes, even warriors get married and if you are, does your spouse have a job? If they do, there is at least a backup source of income should things not go as planned.

Do remember all these points before you quit your day job to do internet marketing full-time. If you do it right, you'll ease smoothly and successfully into being your boss and not working for the man anymore. It's a life-changing event.

Chapter 19. The Biggest Secret To Making Money Online

This one is so obvious yet most beginners don't seem to get it. Here's the secret... **You only make money when you sell.**

That's it. No matter what type of marketing you're doing, you ONLY make money when you sell something. You could be doing affiliate marketing or eCommerce or product creation... Whatever it may be, you still only make money when you sell.

Even for those providing services such as graphic design, content creation, etc. You make money by selling your services.

You must focus on selling! Like they say, "Always be selling."

There's just no getting away from this fact. No amount of learning or buying products and software will ever make you money online if you do not sell. Read that again.

It is so important. You must avoid getting infected with shiny object syndrome.

What's shiny object syndrome?

Shiny object syndrome' is a term commonly used in the internet marketing scene to refer to marketers who keep buying new products that hit the market but never take any action on the info that they buy.

All they seem to do is buy and buy and buy… but they never apply what they learn. They may give some of the methods a try but before anything can gain traction, they quit and start something new.

In the make money online space, thousands of products keep coming out. They have flashy sales pages, sales copy that's hyped up and promises easy profits that will give you the lifestyle of a celebrity rapper.

In reality, most of the products are rehashed and untested theories that just don't work. However, thousands of beginners have to spend a ton of their money on these products and never make a cent in return.

Shiny object syndrome is one of the biggest reasons why most people online fail to make money. They are so busy buying that they never do any selling. The 5 tips below will help you to vaccinate yourself against this 'syndrome' that kills your chances at online success.

Most of it is noise

That's right. Most of the products are released by serial product creators who do not practice what they preach. You need to watch what these marketers are doing instead of what they're saying. The money is in product creation and selling these products.

Forget about the hype and loopholes that their systems promise. If their methods were so good, they'd be doing it themselves but most of them never practice what they preach.

Focus on just one method

Pick a method that is sustainable in the long run. For example, affiliate marketing, eCommerce, etc. Pick just one method and stick to it till you make it work. Only get products related to what you're doing and nothing more.

The method you choose must be a proven business model and not some sneaky loophole that may never work.

Stick to proven products and reputable sellers

Do your research and only buy info products or software that has been proven to work or are created by credible sellers. Ask around for reviews and see if anyone has benefitted from using these products.

The hard truth is that the majority of products have a very short shelf life because they're neither useful nor effective.

Get the right tools only

It's inevitable to reach a point where you need tools to run your online business. You may need membership software, autoresponders, cover creators, etc. Always choose one that is good.

Even if the good ones are a little pricey, you should invest in them. Cheaper alternatives may be unreliable and break down. In some cases, the products may not even deliver what they promise.

So exercise due diligence and stick to proven products that have stood the test of time.

Segment your emails

As a marketer, you'll be inundated with emails from other marketers. All these emails will usually be for offers screaming for your attention. Unsubscribe from lists that offer no value… and for those lists that you are on, do segment the emails to go into separate folders.

You can check them once in a while when you're free. You'll be less tempted to splurge on new products that you don't need.

Other than these 5 tips, do your best not to buy products that you won't use immediately or within a short while. Do not buy

products that you might use 'one day' in the future. In most cases, that one day won't come.

Chapter 20. When The Warrior Fails...

You may have read all the self-help books and the autobiographies of men like Abraham Lincoln who failed all their lives and finally succeeded. It all seems so positive and feel good… until you fail.

One of Mike Tyson's most famous quotes is, *"Everybody has a plan until they get punched in the mouth."*

There's just no denying that failure is a bitter pill to swallow. It doesn't matter how many times you fail, you'll still feel that twinge of disappointment or some anger when your best-laid plans collapse.

Usually, the most successful people are also the ones who are best at coping with failure. The reason for this is that they fail more than most people but they just never give up. That also

means that they do more than most other people who quit the moment failure knocks on their door.

There are many ways to cope with failure but you must understand that it is going to hurt when you fail. Sometimes it may feel like the only thing you ever learn from a failure is that you failed.

While this is not true, it will seem that way. We are all human and no one likes to see their efforts go to waste. It could be a

business venture that collapses. Or maybe your relationship with your spouse crumbles and is beyond repair. Maybe your health takes a turn for the worse despite living a healthy lifestyle.

All of these are events. Understanding this point makes all the difference between handling failure successfully or letting it break you. A failure is an event, not a person.

Like they say, never let success get to your head and never let failure get to your heart. It will hurt and there will be

disappointment… but you must embrace the experience and push forward.

Success is not final and failure is not fatal. As long as you're breathing you still can turn your failures into successes. It's time to discover the 7 secrets that successful people use to cope with failure.

Different individuals may do it differently but the general rule of thumb is this – Failure is always temporary. Failure is not the

opposite of success. It is part of success. Now let's look at how you can cope with it when it comes your way… and you can rest assured that it will. So be prepared.

Don't take it personally.

This is the biggest mistake that most people make. They blame themselves when things go wrong. Or they blame other people. When you do not a separate failure from how you identify yourself, then your self-esteem will drop and you'll be much more tempted to quit.

People usually quit on their dreams because they don't believe that they're capable of achieving what their hearts desire. They feel that it's too hard… and the reason they feel that way is because they may have failed.

For example, when someone is trying to lose weight and watching their diet closely, there will be times when they give in to temptation and eat something they shouldn't. When this

happens, they feel guilt and regret that they failed at maintaining their diet.

What do they do then? They toss their diet aside and gorge themselves on food that they're not supposed to. They believe that they lack the self-discipline to stay focused and lose weight... Just because of one temporary lapse in judgment.

This is ridiculous and it's like accidentally dropping your mobile phone once only to pick it up and keep smashing it on the ground over and over because of one accident. It doesn't make sense... and yet people act similarly.

When you fail at something, whether it's with your blog or your email marketing or if your latest product launch is a flop, do not assume that you're useless and just throw in the towel. What defines you is how well you rise after falling.

So... the most important point to note is that you should not let failure define you as a person. Always know that you can do better.

Learn From Your Mistakes

All the most successful people have learned from their mistakes and try not to repeat them. Failure can also be treated as feedback. If some aspect of your online business fails, ask yourself why this happened.

For example, if your product launch was a flop, there must be a reason why. Was your niche unprofitable? Did the sales page convert poorly? Did you not actively recruit affiliates?

The analysis is very important so that you do not repeat the same errors. This is the only way to make progress and succeed.

Michael Eisner, the Chairman, and CEO of the Disney Corporation said, *"Failure is good as long as it doesn't become a habit."* The only way to prevent failure from becoming a habit is to take stock of your situation, learn from your mistakes and adapt.

Try to maintain a certain degree of detachment so that you can evaluate your failure without feeling bitter. Sometimes it might be a good idea to take a break for a short while and come back to it when you're feeling better. Either way, ALWAYS analyze your failures.

Stop Dwelling On Your Failures

You may have noticed that all some people can talk about is how life has treated them so badly. No matter what they do, they fail at it due to bad luck or unforeseen circumstances.

We've all seen people like these… and while you may not know why these things happen to them, you know that things like these always seem to happen to people like them.

Harsh but very true. Do not dwell on your failures. Analyze them and move on. You have better things in store for you. Missed out on an opportunity? No worries. Better ones are coming your way.

Product launch flopped? That's ok… the next one will sell thousands. Picked the wrong niche to monetize? No big deal. You now know how to find niches with people waiting to buy stuff. Problem solved.

It is inevitable to lose time, effort and money when something

fails. If you keep focusing on what is lost, you'll never be able to focus on what you can gain… and there is so much more out there for you.

Focus on the positive and bury your failures.

Model Other Marketers

There's a saying that you should always learn from the mistakes of others because you'll never live long enough to make them all yourself.

When trying to build an online business, instead of believing all the hype that you see in all the info products that flood the

market, you'd be better off watching what the successful marketers are doing. Do what they do and not what they say.

Most beginners to online marketing encounter failure repeatedly because they follow untested theory and blindly believe what they read or hear. You have to be smarter than that.

If whatever you're doing seems to be failing, then you need to look at what other marketers who are succeeding are doing… then model them. That alone will reduce your learning curve and put you on the path to online success.

Stop being like a housefly that repeatedly bangs its head on the window hoping to get out when the door is wide open for it to go through.

Assess Your Finances

One of the biggest concerns marketers have, when they fail, is that they've lost money. Creating a product costs money. Testing out ads costs money. Outsourcing costs money. There is no getting away from this.

To run any business you need money. It's like oxygen for your business and without it, your business will shrivel up and die. So, you must have a source of income coming in to tide you over if any online endeavor fails.

Some marketers quit their day jobs to make their online business work. When the business fails and the bills start piling up, they start getting desperate.

At times like these, you just may need to get another job to get back on your feet. Do not feel like you have failed and are doomed to a life of 'working for the man.'

This is just a temporary setback… and like Joel Osteen, always

says, "A setback is a set up for a comeback." Go ahead and take that job. It will feel like retrogression but you must understand that even a tiger crouches before it leaps.

Once you have money coming in, the pressure that your finances are causing you will ease. You'll be able to save up some money to keep funding your online business.

That's really how it is. Sometimes you just don't have a choice. Do not throw your efforts down the drain and quit online marketing just because you failed a couple of times. As long as you keep learning and doing, success is inevitable.

Release the Need for Approval from Others.

This is a very common fear and makes failure seem worse than it is. People often worry about what others will think or say about them when they fail. You'll indeed have friends and family members who will tell you, *"I told you so!"* when you fail.

Some of them may even take pleasure in it. This is human nature. It could even be your spouse or parents who don't

support your dreams. When you fail and see their disapproving looks or hear their sarcastic words, it can seem worse.

The truth of the matter is that you only have one life to live and you need to live it for yourself. It doesn't matter what others say or think about you. Just because others think you're dumb for failing doesn't mean that you're foolish.

How people see you should have zero impact on how you see yourself. Have faith in yourself and don't pay heed to the naysayers.

Take a Break

Time heals all wounds. Sometimes when failure gets to you, it may be time to take a break and put some space between you and your business. This will help to clear your mind so that you can think objectively.

While taking a break, you can self-reflect and think about your plans. You may decide to have backup plans to correct any future failures or problems that may crop up.

Take the time to exercise. Research has shown that hard training like boxing, Crossfit, sprinting, etc. helps people to release pent up frustration and anger.

This can be therapeutic when coping with failure. Instead of hitting the bottle, you can hit a punching bag or lift heavy weights explosively during CrossFit sessions. Do what suits you best.

What is most important is that you not let failure make you quit. That is the most common consequence of failure. People fail a few times and they quit.

If you read the story of Colonel Sanders, you'd realize that he was turned down 1,009 times before he finally found someone who would use his recipe. Walt Disney was turned down over 300 times before he received financing for Disney World.

By any standards, you could say that these guys were massive failures… **Until they succeeded**. The difference is that they kept going while the masses would have quit long ago. *Would you keep going if you failed 1,009 times?*

How about 10 times? Most people don't even get past 2 failures. So what if you fail? It's no big deal. You get up, dust yourself and move on. That's the only way to succeed… To keep on keeping on. You can do it.

"I've missed more than 9000 shots in my career. I've lost almost 300 games. 26 times, I've been trusted to take the game-winning shot and missed. I've failed over and over and over again in my life. And that is why I succeed." - **Michael Jordan**

Chapter 21 . What It All Comes Down To

This is a quote by Leonardo da Vinci – "Simplicity is the ultimate sophistication."

It's a fantastic quote that should apply all aspects of your life, especially so when building an online business. Most people make internet marketing more difficult than it is.

The buy so many products and so much software that they get overwhelmed. Their computer desktop is cluttered with icons and their business is a mess because it's all so chaotic.

Many beginners are also held back from progressing because of their tendency to overcomplicate things. They make the process harder than it is and then feel like it's all too hard for them.

Keep your business simple and it will be successful. It's not difficult to do this.

Be organized

This is the first step to simplicity. Plan your day so that you know exactly what tasks to do for that day. Make sure the folders on your computer are well-organized and easy to find.

Keep the most important and often used files on your desktop and clear the rest away into some other folder that's not on your screen.

Get an external storage drive to save all files that you just need to keep as a record. This will save space on your computer and speed things up.

Master the fundamentals

You must master the basics before moving on to more complex tasks. If you do not know the basics of video creation, don't buy the most expensive and complex video editing software that you can find and struggle to figure it out.

Spend time learning the basics until you understand the terminology and the different aspects of video creation. Once you have a firm grasp of the fundamentals, you can take on more complex tasks.

Stick to the basics

Some people work best with a pen and paper. Some use planners. Others use software like Trello online to stay organized. You just need to use what you're most comfortable with.

If you find it easier to just scribble notes on paper, then do that. Even if it's basic and not all 'techy'… if it works for you, stick to it. There's no need to master Trello or Evernote just because everyone else is using these. Do what suits you best.

Always have a backup plan

You should do your best to have a Plan B whenever possible. For example, if you're quitting your day job to do online marketing full time, make sure you have at least enough savings to tide you for six months in case of any unforeseen circumstances.

If you blindly quit your day job and your online business does not take off, the financial stress is going to affect you and take a toll on you mentally and emotionally. You'll be working from a place of desperation.

Keep things simple and plan well in advance.

Stay grounded

When you do succeed online, you'll be tempted to get a bigger house or a better car or more expensive things now that you can afford it. While the occasional reward is good for the soul, do not overdo it.

If you buy a flashy car with high monthly payments that require you to work crazy hours online just to keep up, then you don't own the car. The car owns you.

The same can be said for any material possession that causes you stress because you need to constantly work hard to afford it.

Live within your means. Do not fall into the trap of buying things you don't need with money that you don't have, to impress people who don't care. It's unnecessary stress.

Keep things as simple as possible in all aspects of your life.

"The cost of a thing is the amount of what I will call life which is

required to be exchanged for it, immediately or in the long run." - Henry David Thoreau

Chapter 22. Be A Warrior, Not a Worrier

You've reached the end of this book. If you're still reading this, you've done better than most who would have quit halfway.

Now, all you need to do is apply what you've read. While the info in this guide may seem simple, that doesn't make it easy. You'll need to dig deep to keep going when things get hard.

Do reread this book whenever the need arises. Cast your worries aside and have faith in yourself. Aim for balance in your life.

Know with resolute confidence that you'll reach your goals.

Once you have faith in yourself, then it's just a matter of putting one foot in front of another and carrying on. There will be no need to rush or feel fear. You're going to reach your destination no matter what.

As long as you take action and do what you need to, you'll truly become a warrior marketer. You'll have your health, your fitness, a super cool body, a successful online business and the knowledge that you did it all without letting anything slide.

This is priceless. Weapons and situations may change... but warriors don't. Stay true to what you learned from this book and you'll be unbeatable.

Chapter 23. The Aim – What it Takes to be a Warrior

So, what are the tenants of the warrior mindset? What words can we use to describe the modern warrior? Here are just a few:

- **Courageous**
- **Self-Disciplined**
- **Principled**
- **Strong-willed**
- **Kind**
- **Growth-oriented**
- **Self-sufficiency**
- **Protective**
- **Self-Sacrificing**
- **Calm**
- **Responsible**
- **Motivational, Inspiring, Charismatic**
- **Noble**
- **Powerful**
- **Modest (though not necessarily humble)**

These are just some of the traits that a true warrior should strive for. These are some of the things we will be looking to cultivate and better understand throughout this book.

Another great description of a warrior comes from an unlikely source: the Disney film *Mulan*. These quotes are from the song 'I'll Make a Man Out of You' but in fact, they can apply equally to a woman.

Oh, and in case you don't want to learn lessons on chivalry from a Disney film, consider the fact that Jackie Chan sang the Chinese version of the song. He's one of life's true warriors, so perhaps that gives it just a little more weight…

Tranquil as a forest But on fire within.

Once you find your center You are sure to win.

We must be swift as a coursing river with all the force of a great typhoon With all the strength of a raging fire Mysterious as the dark side of the moon.

Still and calm on the outside then, but with great power and strength on the inside. Not driven by impulse or whim, but by a greater purpose. Never bending to the will of others and never giving up when the going gets tough. That is the warrior spirit.

Chapter 24. Times You Were Not a Warrior

You probably don't live on the battlefield and you probably *hopefully* will never need to see combat (although this book will ensure that you are ready in case you ever do).

But there are plenty of ways that the warrior mindset will apply in your day-to-day life as well and plenty of opportunities to demonstrate what it takes to be a warrior.

Perhaps the easiest way to consider this is to look at all those times that you *weren't* a warrior in your life. These are the times when your fear, your anger or your lack of motivation and willpower got the better of you.

Consider this:

You wake up in the morning and realize your favorite shirt is torn, you spend the rest of the day angry with everyone, sulking and not focussing on your work. This very small inconvenience has ruined your ability to stay productive and it has made other people feel bad.

It's raining out so you call off your plans to visit your friend down the road, who you know was looking forward to the get-together.

You're trying to lose weight but you're low on energy and so you eat a large piece of cake.

A friend faints at a party and instead of staying calm and following a correct protocol to make sure they're okay, you instead get in a flap, scream at everyone and make matters worse.

Your boss needs you to complete an assignment before you go home. You resent the idea of staying later and you're feeling tired so you rush it and put in less than your best work.

You have been telling friends for years that you're going to write a book and that it is your dream to become a published author. You get home and the first thing you do is crash on the couch and watch trashy TV.

You break a glass in the kitchen and when your partner asks who did it, you blame your friend who was round the other day.

You get into a physical altercation with someone in the street and run away – leaving your friends or family to deal with the danger on their own.

You are getting onto a train and instead of letting the elderly lady on in front of you, you push ahead.

Your friends are peer pressuring you into smoking weed and accusing you of not being fun. Smoking weed is something you have no interest in this hypothetical situation but you let yourself get talked into it for fear of appearing lame.

You are happily married when an attractive woman/man makes their move on you. You give in to your momentary impulse and you sleep with them, effectively wrecking your relationship with not only your partner but your children as well.

You are unhappy in your relationship or job but you stay in it because you don't have the heart to tell the person or you are too afraid of what the future might bring.

Some of these examples are more extreme than others. Of course, there is a big difference between eating ice cream when you really shouldn't and being swayed by hate speech! And occasionally losing your cool is normal. But while these points might all seem very different, they essentially come from the same thing: weakness.

Weakness is often the source of our problems and even of evil. Weakness means giving in to things we know aren't right, or making excuses and putting off our goals.

Now let's look at how someone *strong* might approach the same issues:

You wake up in the morning and realize your favorite shirt is torn. You shrug and wear something else, recognizing this is a very small issue in the grand scheme of things!

It's raining out and you don't feel like going out. But you know it's the right thing to do, so you man up and you go.

You're trying to lose weight but you're low on energy. You dig deep, find that fire within and head to the gym.

A friend faints at a party and you remain calm, cool and collected. You assign jobs to people and check they're okay.

Your boss needs you to complete an assignment before you go home. You resent the idea of staying later and you're feeling tired but you complete the work to the best of your ability nevertheless. You speak to your boss about not putting you in that position again.

You have been telling friends for years that you're going to write a book and that it is your dream to become a published author. You get home and resolve to write two pages a night.

You break a glass in the kitchen and when your partner asks who did it, you own up and face the consequences.

You get into a physical altercation with someone in the street. You make sure your family and friends are safe while trying to calm the situation as best you can.

You are getting onto a train and you *always* stop to let the old lady on first. And the old man. And anyone who was there first.

Your friends are peer pressuring you into smoking weed and accusing you of not being fun. If you want to, you do it. If you do not, you do not.

You are happily married when an attractive woman/man makes their move on you. You have control of your feelings so you turn them down.

You are unhappy in your relationship or job so you discuss that unhappiness with the other party and look for ways to improve the situation. That might mean finding a new job or ending the relationship but it is better than dragging it out.

The warrior is mentally and physically strong and this allows them to stick to their code of ethics and to work toward their vision for a better future – instead of doing what makes them feel good in the short term.

Ultimately, this leads to much greater happiness, much greater peace and much greater pride. And not just for you, but for all those around you.

Chapter 25. The Fire Within

That line, the 'fire within' is one that speaks great volumes about the warrior mindset. And it calls to mind lyrics from another song: 'Hearts On Fire' by the (excellent) band Survivor.

A great line from that song goes:

In the warrior's code, there's no surrender Though his body says stop, his spirit cries: "Never!"

So, what is this telling us about the warrior mentality? Simple: warriors don't give up and they don't give in.

(I also enjoy Vegeta's line: *you may have invaded my mind and body but there's one thing a Saiyan always keeps… his pride!*)

So how do you gain this kind of iron will and determination? How do you develop the unstoppable ability to *never give up*?

It starts by knowing what you want to achieve and by having a set of principles.

To use *yet another* quote, Alice Cooper and Xzibit sang:

If you don't stand for something, you will fall for anything

And this is completely true. If you have no specific goal and no set of values that is entirely your own, then how can you be expected to stick rigidly to those values?

If you haven't defined who you are, what you're about and what is important to you, then, of course, it will be easy to get tempted by good food, trashy TV or other 'easy options'. Of course, it will be easy for you to be swayed by the influence and the politics of others.

Moreover, having a goal is what will give you the motivation and the energy to get up and work toward the things you are truly excited about.

Think about someone like Arnold Schwarzenegger or Dwayne Johnson. These are people who have accomplished incredible things and part of the reason for that is undoubtedly their seemingly endless energy. Their ability to get up every single day and know what they want to do.

Can you *imagine* seeing the Rock look tired and dejected? Have you ever seen Arnold Schwarzenegger look indifferent or bored?

These people have tireless energy but it comes from a vision and a goal. And so it is with *all* the most accomplished people throughout history.

Arnie said this of his burning desire and how it led him to accomplish his goals:

With my desire and drive, I wasn't normal. Normal people can be happy with a regular life. I was different. I felt there was more to life than plodding through a normal existence... I have always been impressed by stories of greatness and power. I wanted to do something special, to be recognized as the best. I saw bodybuilding as the vehicle that would take me to the top, and I put all my energy into it.

The point is: knowing what you want from life will fuel you with energy, whether that is wanting what's best for your family, wanting to achieve creative accomplishments, wanting to reach a certain point in your career... etc.

Think about a new parent. Parents have seemingly endless energy and will sacrifice their sleep, their finances, and their happiness to look after their children. They can accomplish anything because they have found something greater than themselves.

A parent's love will give them that warrior's mindset but you can't rely on just that. To accomplish the most and to build the best world for your family and friends, you also need something that is *intrinsically* motivating to you.

In other words, you need a purpose and a goal that doesn't rely on anyone else – so that even when no one needs you, you still have the strength to pull yourself out of bed and to refuse distractions and unhelpful desires.

Once you have your goal, you will find a passion. And once you have a passion you will find that you have endless energy and drive and that you even speak with more conviction and greater charisma.

Did you know that we gesticulate more when we speak about something that we're passionate about? That's because we are now speaking with our entire bodies – our body language is congruent with what we are saying.

And did you know that when people see us speak in that way, they rate us as more charismatic? More inspiring? And better leaders?

When we believe in what we are saying, we will be more efficient at getting *others* to believe it. This is how movements are started and this makes us far more attractive and magnetic.

And with your goal and your objective, you will better be able to make decisions and to avoid unnecessary distractions. You will be more decisive and you will be more impressive. Why? Because you can consider every decision through the following lens: 'does this help me to achieve my goals'? If the answer is no, then you do something else.

What career path should you take? The one that helps you to achieve your overarching goals. What party should you vote for? The one that helps you to fulfill your vision.

The point of the goal is to have something greater than yourself – something worth fighting for.

This single-mindedness was central to the psychology of all of history's greatest warriors, though it took a very different form. Historically, you had your samurai and your knights. A samurai's training went to great measures to ensure their loyalty to a 'shogun' (a master samurai). They would be willing to die for their shogun, just as a king's knight would be willing to die for king and country.

Today though, this is dangerous thinking. We are all too aware that our politicians are flawed and we've seen how blindly following a leader or a set of beliefs can lead to terrible atrocities.

So, what we need to do instead is to create our own set of values and principles. Rules to live by and a goal or a vision to strive for. This can change but we must never let others force us to act against our code.

Unfortunately, there is no objectively 'correct' way to approach life. We don't know why reality exists, what is waiting for us on the other side (if anything) or what the meaning of life is. Therefore, it is up to each of us to make our way by assessing our values, principles, and rules to live by.

Chapter 26. Finding Your Goal

So, let us start with finding a goal, something greater than yourself to strive toward. A purpose that you will be an instrument in accomplishing.

So this might mean that you set about changing the world for the better.

Maybe you want to put an end to world

hunger, maybe you want to help slow down global warming, or perhaps you are interested in becoming a rock star or a musician. Maybe you just want to get rich.

No goal is 'wrong', it is simply having a goal and something to be passionate about that will give you the fuel and the fire to keep going no matter what.

Goals *start* with visions. To visualize the way you want life to be 5 or 10 years for now. Picture where you are, what your surroundings are, who you are with, what you've accomplished. This should be a vision that makes you excited and energized – your perfect life. For inspiration, consider the times in your life you were happiest, consider what you wanted to be as a child and picture some of your role models and what you can perhaps learn from them.

This is what you will picture to drive yourself toward change and greatness.

This is what will get you out of bed in the morning. And then on top of that, you are going to structure yourself goals – smaller, more measurable steps that will help you to reach that point.

Chapter 27. Creating Your Own Code of Ethics

On top of this, you will build your code of ethics. Your idea of what you consider to be 'living well' and 'doing the right thing'.

Again, this doesn't have to be your conventional set of rules. It might be that you don't agree with some aspects of the law. Some well-known philosophers are known for views that stray from conventional ideas about ethics and morality.

Take Ayn Rand for example, who believed that morality comes from what makes them happiest. She said:

Man has no automatic code of survival…. His senses do not tell him automatically what is good for him or evil, what will benefit his life or endanger it, what goals he should pursue and what means will achieve them, what values his life depends on, what course of action it requires. Man must choose his actions, values, and goals by the standard of that which is proper to man - to achieve, maintain, fulfill and enjoy that ultimate value, that end in itself, which is his own life.

She believed that individual morality should be based on what makes that individual happiest. That means working on things that you love, improving yourself and protecting the ones you care about… who in turn make you happier.

Rand would suggest that we should look after our families and our loved ones, pursue our passions and our self-betterment and that way contribute to society.

Whatever *you* believe your code to be, you write it down and then commit to sticking to that code. That way, you won't be persuaded by other people, you will be able to fight for your values and people will know where they stand with you.

That said, you also shouldn't be afraid to evolve and adapt your ideas over time. That is why it is so important to keep reading and keep learning. Keep up to date with politics and what is going on in the world, read philosophy and reassess your values.

There is no value in sticking to one set of goals or principles indefinitely and refusing to readdress them, as ultimately this becomes a 'lie' as much as any other

You should not vote a certain way because you have always voted a certain way. And you should not be afraid to reassess the way that you feel about certain aspects of your code.

The point is that you will not break your code of conduct while it exists. You have standards to uphold and the simple act of upholding them will make you a stronger, braver and more impressive individual.

And note that in the ideal scenario, there should be some interplay between what you believe, your code of ethics, your goals and your political views. Hopefully, you have a vision for where you think the world should go, what you think life should be like. Your goals are there to help you achieve that, while your code of ethics should also ensure that you don't miss the trees for the forest.

All this results in you becoming a person who knows what they believe and who knows themselves. And when you know that, you will be a greater and more powerful individual.

Chapter 28. Overcoming Fear

When we think of the archetypal warrior, we will almost certainly be sure to think of someone brave, courageous and seemingly fearless. This is the kind of person that will walk into the line of fire. That will speak out against injustice, that will take on enemies that are much greater than them.

In our personal lives, there are no real dragons to slay. Rather, they take on many other forms, whether they be illness, whether they be debt, or whether they be the struggle of going to the gym every day…

If you're a fan of reading self-help literature then chances are that at some point you will have written down your goals. This is something that almost every guru seems to advise and that many claims can help you to accomplish your dreams by better defining and visualizing them.

But in Tim Ferriss' *4 Hour Workweek* this advice is turned on its head somewhat. While Tim doesn't necessarily have a problem with goal setting per-say, he also recommends doing essentially the opposite by 'fear setting'. And he claims it can do a great deal more than goal setting when it comes to realizing your aims and getting more from life…

What is Fear Setting?

The general idea behind fear setting is that you're defining the fears that are holding you back so that you can face them. In most cases, Tim postulates that after doing this you'll find that your fears are actually relatively unfounded and thus

will move forward and past them. Normally our fears are of 'irreversible' negative outcomes, but actually, these are rarer than you might think…

So what you do is to write down the absolute worst possible outcomes for doing whatever it is you want to do, and then write down all the ways you'd cope with the situation or possibly reverse it.

An Example: Changing Career

Let's take a changing career as an example. This is something that a lot of people want to do, but feel held back by fear of the potential repercussions. By defining those fears though, you can minimize their potency.

So if you were going to write down the worst possible outcomes for changing careers, it might well look something like this:

I might leave my job only to fail to find another job.

I might be unable to pay the mortgage and thus be forced to move home.

This could upset my partner so much they leave me.

I might get the job I think I want and find out I hate it more than my last job

I might apply to other jobs only to get rejected by everyone and end up damaging my ego.

These are all real concerns, but now if you think about all the ways you can manage risk and reduce the impacts of those negative outcomes you'll find your fears aren't all that founded…

I can look for jobs without leaving my current job to avoid the risk of unemployment. No one has to know.

This will also be a lot less reckless in the eyes of my partner.

Alternatively, I could speak to my boss about my problems and see if there are other positions within my organization.

If I do end up out of work I could always speak to my old boss about getting my job back/work in a supermarket while I look for other work/work for Dad/live off of savings for a couple of months/move back home with the parents!

If my partner leaves me for trying to become happier then I need to reassess that relationship.

If I don't like the job I find next then I will feel more confident about job hunting again in the future.

If I struggle to get accepted by anywhere I can work on my interview technique/improve my CV/seek career guidance. All of which will be useful experiences anyway.

As you can see then, the very worst scenario is probably not as bad as it seems – it may just mean living out of savings for a while or taking a small step backward to take two forwards. Likewise, as there are so many ways to minimize the risk of things going wrong, it's quite unlikely you'll end up in those positions anyway.

In *The 4 Hour Workweek* Tim also gives one other piece of advice that I feel is very relevant here: don't ask for permission, ask for forgiveness. Take that attitude and outline your fears and you're on track to a happier version of yourself as well as to accomplish much more.

Chapter 30. Stoicism and the Warrior Mindset

Tim Ferriss' ideas might seem unique but actually, he says that he is inspired by ancient philosophy and specifically, by the ideas of the ancient Stoics. Stoicism is a school of philosophy the way back to the 3rd Century BC. Its principles were founded and practiced by historical characters such as Epictetus, Seneca and Marcus Aurelius.

And in many ways, Stoicism was an early approach to a 'warrior mindset'. It was all about mental hardiness and about learning to expect and then live with things going wrong. Many of us describe someone brave and courageous as *being stoic*.

So, what precisely does it involve?

The Power of Pessimism

If we tell someone that we don't think things are going to work out as we hoped, then they'll often tell us that we need to be 'more optimistic'.

There's even a song that tells us to 'accentuate the positive' and 'eliminate the negative'. The consensus is clear: being positive is a good thing and being anything *other* than positive is unacceptable.

But is this the best way for us to approach our problems? Or is it perhaps actually quite *damaging* to constantly be blinded by optimism? Does it leave us vulnerable to disappointment and potentially easily caught off guard? Is expected life to be constantly 'sunshine and rainbows' the precise opposite of a warrior mindset?

Wouldn't a warrior accept and embrace the fact that life is going to be hard? And then toughen themselves up to deal with it?

That's the view held by stoics at least and when you delve into the philosophy a little, you might find that they make a very good case for pessimism.

The Central Ideas of Stoicism

The general gist of stoicism is not to try and 'shut out' negativity and pretend that bad thing doesn't happen but rather to *embrace* it and even to use it as a tool. *Hope,* according to the stoics, is the enemy, precisely because it means we're unprepared for things going wrong and we're likely to be disappointed.

Instead, stoicism advocates the notion of gritty realism – of recognizing the negative aspects of life and accepting that a lot of what happens is out of our control and is probably not going to be very pleasant!

Using Stoicism in Your Own Life

This might not sound like a particularly helpful stance to take on things, but then that's because most of us are highly trained into only accepting positive viewpoints. This is the general conceit of countless self-help books and even Hollywood films. Dream big and you can get what you want! It's pretty much the driving force behind capitalism.

But the Stoics take the opposite approach. They prepare for the storm. They learn to enjoy life even when things aren't going their way and they recognize hardship as challenge and an opportunity for growth.

When you go through life feeling *entitled* to everything going your way, how can you expect to be happy? And how can you be expected to face genuinely difficult challenges?

So how does rejecting this incessant positivity help? How do you practically apply stoicism in your own life?

Negative Visualization

One suggestion from stoicism is something called 'negative visualization' – the idea that you visualize your fears rather than your goals. Instead of picturing things going perfectly to plan, instead, picture things at their very worst. Imagine how your plans can fail and picture what life would be like if all of your worst fears came true.

What this does is to first help you to prepare for those worst-case scenarios. Once you know what your fears look like, you can then think about how you would cope in that scenario. Often, you'll find that this worst-case scenario is not as bad as you at first thought it would be. And in other cases, you'll find that you can find ways to cope with that situation.

This removes fears that could otherwise hold you back *and* means that you aren't blindly ignoring what could potentially go wrong.

If this sounds familiar then that's because it's precisely the same concept that helped Tim Ferriss to come up with his Fear Setting technique.

Be Content With the Scantiest and Cheapest Fare

In one of his letters to Lucilius, Seneca said:

Set aside a certain number of days, during which you shall be content with the scantiest and cheapest fare, with the coarse and rough dress, saying to yourself the while: is this the condition that I feared?

The general idea here is that you should not only visualize your worst-case scenario but also try *living* it. That might mean spending a week living off of minimum salary, it might even mean sleeping rough.

In either case, this teaches you not only that you can handle your worst fears – and therefore have less reason to be afraid – but also that you don't *need* material possessions to be happy.

This is very important to cultivate. It takes great discipline to part with your possessions and belongings but the result is freedom from fear and also from many physical restrictions. If you are weighed down by possessions and belongings, then you will not be able to move home freely. You will spend a lot of time cleaning and attending to things that *do not* help you further your goals. And ultimately, you will have much more to fear.

The more you own, the more you have to lose. This creates a sense of fear.

So, try to declutter and live a more focussed and minimalist life. At the very least, learn to detach yourself from physical possessions and remember that they are true 'just things'. They are a means to an end and if you must sacrifice them, so be it.

Selling your widescreen TV or turning down a holiday to pay off debt or pay for your child's tuition – those are warrior-like choices.

Wear Ugly Clothes…

Another classic stoic move is to wear 'ugly' clothes to teach yourself not to be ashamed. People might stare at you, but this will simply teach you that it doesn't matter at all what others think – only what *you think.*

This is an important aspect of the warrior

mindset: caring what other people think makes you vulnerable to peer pressure and vanity. Sometimes, to do what must be done, you must be willing to sacrifice your reputation.

Just as in our example about admitting that you broke the vase…

Expect the Worst

Stoics argue that we curse when we're angry and that this anger is our failing – our stupidity.

Think about the last time you swore with anger. Chances are that it was not because it rained or because you found you were in debt. More likely, it was

because you dropped something on your toe, or because you broke your favorite possession.

The point is that the anger comes from the *surprise*, not the disappointment. You don't swear when it rains because you know that rain is a possibility.

Therefore, if you are angry, this then suggests that you didn't expect whatever happened to you and this is arguably *your fault*. If you accept that bad things happen and if you accept that sometimes things won't go to plan, then you will not need to be angry – because you will have accounted for it and prepared mentally for it.

Now, when your partner cheats on you, or when a service provider doesn't deliver a good service, you will think of it as being simply a part of life – just like the rain.

Control Your Reaction

Stoicism means submitting to the fact that you have scant-to-no control over reality. But at the same time, it also means taking solace in the knowledge that these outside factors can't hurt you – only your reaction can.

You can't control what happens to you but you can control what *you* make of that event and your interpretation of it. Being mentally prepared for things that could go wrong is one good example of this in action. Likewise, though, you might also simply decide not to let things affect you – to take a step back from

them and to deal with the consequences rather than thrashing against things that you cannot change.

This is something we'll be addressing more closely in upcoming chapters: mindfulness and the ability to decide how *you* want to react to the things going on around you.

But simply by remembering that tough things happen and it's your job to deal with them, you should find you can

I think that Rocky Balboa is one of the great modern stoics – and one of his more recent famous quotes summarises the ideas of Seneca and Marcus Aurelius perfectly:

The world ain't all sunshine and rainbows. It's a very mean and nasty place... and I don´t care how tough you are, it will beat you to your knees and keep you there permanently if you let it. You, me or nobody, is gonna hit as hard as life. But ain't about how hard you hit... It's about how hard you can get hit, and keep moving forward... how much you can take, and keep moving forward. That´s how winning is done.

Here's a quote from fiction a book *I* wrote several years ago. This line was spoken by a reckless character in the story and was never meant to carry much weight. But I found that as I thought about it, it was surprisingly true:

Those that fear death, fear life.

It is true that if you live life in fear of death, then you will be permanently cautious. You will not take risks and you will not live life to its fullest as a result.

So, what is the solution? Do we put death 'out of our mind'?

No: it would be better to come to terms with it and stoically, simply accept it as a reality. And this mirrors the way that the Samurai would approach their lives too. Here is a quote from Edo samurai DaidojiYuzan, which can be found in the book *Code of the Samurai*:

One who is a samurai must before all things keep constantly in mind…the fact that he has to die. If he is always mindful of this, he will be able to live following the paths of loyalty and filial duty, will avoid myriads of evils and adversities, keep himself free of disease and calamity and moreover enjoy a long life.

He will also be a fine personality with many admirable qualities.

For existence is impermanent as the dew of evening, and the hoarfrost of morning, and particularly uncertain is the life of the warrior…

Remember your goals and your vision. Work toward them. Stick to your code. Try to make a difference and focus on what you leave behind.

That might mean protecting your family even when it means putting yourself at risk, or it might mean taking chances to chase after a bigger goal.

Chapter 31. Growth Mindset

In the last chapter, we looked at the importance of overcoming fear – even overcoming a fear of death.

And similarly, it is equally important to be willing to be uncomfortable and to experience small amounts of hardship. How can you lose weight if you are afraid of dieting? How can you expect to progress in your career if you shy away from hard work?

But this is the reality for many of us. We are simply unwilling to do things we don't want to do or to put up with hard times. We have become exceedingly weak and it is ultimately making us unhappy.

Consider your dog and compare them to a wolf (if you don't own a dog, consider the one you know). Look at the differences.

Your dog might be loving, loyal and fun but it is entirely dependent on you. It wouldn't survive a day in the wild and it's certainly not a *warrior* like a wolf is.

Why not? Because it has been domesticated. And that my friend, is your problem as well.

We have not only become domesticated but we have also become lazy, spoiled and overly indulged. In modern society, everything is disposable, everything comes easily and we never have to wait.

Hungry? Order a takeaway. It will be with you in five minutes and it will be packed with salt and sugar so you feel a rush of reward hormones.

Horny? Watch some porn.

Bored? Turn on the TV and laugh at someone falling over. Need information? Just ask Siri.

Want to get into better shape? Naah, that seems like a lot of effort.

Being so constantly indulged in whatever we want means that we find it harder than ever to put in the effort when it is needed. Why *would* we put in the effort when we can have so much, so easily?

And likewise, when we are used to getting whatever we want, we feel distraught when the shower doesn't heat up properly.

And here's the thing: in the wild, you would have *only* had cold water to wash in. Eating would have required hunting or foraging in the rain while avoiding predators. You could be so much stronger and so much tougher – mentally *and* physically. But as we are, we're fat, lazy and low on motivation.

Chapter 32. How to Get Tough

So with that in mind, how do you go about getting tough?

The first thing you need to do is to try living with less. We discussed this already in our post on Stoicism, but traveling is a fantastic way to accomplish the warrior mindset. That means traveling and staying in hostels, not booking hotels the night before, only taking a few clothes.

I have been on a few journeys like this myself.

I went on a trip around Europe and took only a backpack to get by. I remember lying at a train station in Poland in the snow, unable to read the signposts (despite my Polish heritage) and not knowing when the next train would come.

Or even where I was! This was before data roaming or 3G, so that was out of the question too.

Then I found a little cafe and managed to order some tea – with milk rather than with a lemon as the Polish generally drink it.

You know what? I felt bliss drinking from that polystyrene cup. I appreciated the tea *so much* because it had been so long and because I was so cold.

Today, I often ask for my tea in polystyrene cups when it's an option because it sends me back to that moment.

And this is what you realize when you force yourself to do without you learn that the little things can bring you a lot of joy. That there are rewards and happiness to be found in every moment. You don't *need* everything to go perfectly.

And, when things go wrong, it creates stories and helps you to grow stronger.

And that's a key point actually: to keep a growth mindset at all times. Each challenge that comes your way is a chance to get stronger, smarter and better. By dealing with these hardships, your life has a greater purpose (life is meaningless when it is easy) and you become better equipped to take on similar challenges in the future.

So, the next time you find yourself in debt, instead of letting it defeat you, instead see it as a challenge. How can you earn the money you need to get out of it? How can you become *better*?

Don't wallow in stress or anxiety – that helps no one.

See it as a chance to grow and to prevent this from happening again and take the necessary steps. Don't worry about how it looks to others, don't blame yourself for letting yourself get into that situation before.

Just take action. And learn from it. You were not good enough before but now you are going to be better.

Growth and challenges are things that the brain is *wired for*. We *thrive* when we are challenged mentally and physically and this results in the production of hormones like dopamine, brain-derived neurotrophic factor and more that keep us focussed and that help protect our brains into old age.

Not only should you welcome the challenges that come, but you should also seek them out.

During 'times of peace', you should prepare for battle by learning (reading books, adopting new skills) and by training your body.

Tools for Growth and Resilience

We've talked a lot about how the warrior mindset involves greater resilience, greater patience, calmness, and strength. But the real question is how you get to that point. How can you *gain* that warrior mindset?

Hopefully, by now, you understand what the warrior mindset *is* and what it means in a broader context but how can you overcome your weaknesses and your urge to eat cake, to relax and to take the easy options?

Here are a few powerful tools that will help you to grow and become stronger.

Chapter 33. Correct Breathing

Another tool you can use to regain your composure and enter the warrior mindset at will is correct breathing. This means belly breathing, breathing from your diaphragm first and taking deep breaths. This calms your nervous system and puts you into the rest and digest state, it's the perfect way to overcome anxiety.

Cold showers increase your metabolism, they help you produce more testosterone and they cause a flood of adrenaline. They can strengthen your immune system too. In other words, they're good for you and a great way to start your day.

But at the same time, they hurt and they suck. This is a terrible shock to the system and it's the last thing you want to do.

Which is *precisely* why it is ideal for your warrior training. Taking cold showers requires incredible mental discipline and if you can force yourself to do this every day, then you can achieve just about anything.

And as a fun fact, Hugh Jackman said that he used cold showers as a way to get into the mind of Wolverine for the X-Men movies.

Now there's a warrior that you could afford to be more like!

Chapter 35. Strength Training and Martial Arts

What do all the warriors through history have in common?

They are not just mentally tough – although that has been the focus of this book – they are also physically tough. This is very important because physical toughness gives you the strength, the resolve and the power to be confident and to make a stand when you *do* need to fight for your values.

It is important where possible not to fight but actually, being formidable physically will help you to avoid the *need* to fight.

Not only that, but it will give you the ability to protect the ones you love.

And both martial arts and weight lifting will help you to grow while also instilling *great* self-discipline. To increase your chances of succeeding on your journey, take up a martial art and endeavor to hit the gym 3 or 4 times a week.

As Socrates said:

No man has the right to be an amateur in the matter of physical training. It is a shame for a man to grow old without seeing the beauty and strength of which his body is capable.

Chapter 36. Applying Classic Warrior Principles to Business and Life

I always thought it was something of a fashion statement for businessmen and women to carry copies of *The Art of War* by Sun Tsu. I understood their claim that it was relevant to business strategy and that many of the ideas are still relevant, but it all seemed a bit fanciful to me.

More like vanity and posing! How could a thousand-year-old treatise genuinely be relevant to today's world of computers and mobile phones?

That was until I began to practice the warrior mindset and quickly realized that it *is* highly relevant. Sure, it won't teach you to use MSWord, but in terms of marketing, leadership and the management of resources it is still very useful.

These ideas and suggestions are timeless and can be applied in almost limitless situations.

Look at it this way, if the advice is good enough to help you win wars with swords and arrows, then surely it can help you to get Bill from accounting to stop complaining.

With that in mind, I present some of the best quotes and lessons from the book that you can take with you into the office and us to inspire more loyalty and productivity. And just for good measure, I've thrown in some Machiavelli; who wrote *The Prince* as an instruction manual for an Italian prince that would help him to become an effective ruler someday.

These are both texts aimed at historical warriors and kings and yet they are covered by business professionals, relationship gurus and more. This is the *perfect* example of why the warrior mindset is still relevant today and you will see that the sentiments therein echo much of what we have already discussed.

Chapter 37. Lessons from the Art of War

There is No Instance of a Nation Benefiting From Prolonged Warfare

In other words, if you are at odds with a competitor or a colleague then a prolonged struggle will only serve to damage *both* of you. This is called a 'pyrrhic victory' – a phrase that comes from another famous historical battle. By the end even if you win, you will have damaged your

reputation and wasted your resources so that you're left with nothing but a Pyrrhic Victory. Instead, then, see if you can't turn an opponent into an ally and find a way that you both can benefit instead.

Remember, the warrior chooses their battles wisely. The warrior mindset is not about being aggressive and reactionary. It is about being poised, forgiving and powerful enough to *not need* to lift a finger.

This then explains another of Sun Tsu's quotes: *the supreme art of war is to subdue the enemy without fighting.* This is *highly* relevant to modern warriors – truer now than ever before.

Opportunities Multiply As They Are Seized

If you wanted an example of how The Art of War can directly apply to business then this is it. How much more perfect could you want this to describe the process of making investments? You have to spend to accumulate!

Remember how Arnie chose bodybuilding as a path and a springboard to greater success? You can similarly choose wisely to yield incredible results from simple starting points.

Know the enemy and know yourself; in a hundred battles, you will never be in peril.

This is an obvious one that rams home the importance of both researching the market, and looking at your feedback to ensure you are best prepared to take on the competition.

In case you thought Sun Tsu only glosses over obvious points though he goes on to expand: *When you are ignorant of the enemy, but know yourself, your chances of winning or losing are equal. If ignorant of both your enemy and yourself, you are certain in every battle to be in peril.*

Outside of the office, we have already discussed how knowing yourself will allow you to form your own rules and your own goals and objectives.

The general who advances without coveting fame and retreats without fearing disgrace, whose only thought is to protect his country and do good service for his sovereign, is the jewel of the kingdom.

This is the kind of employee you want - keep an eye on those who bring too much ego to the workplace. This is the kind of employee you need to be. And this perfectly echoes Seneca's views on living with less earlier on.

Remember, in this case, you are not serving your country or sovereign but the higher purpose and values that *you chose for yourself.*

Victorious warriors win first and then go to war, while defeated warriors go to war first and then seek to win.

Planning is *everything*. Before you bring your product or service to market your success or failure is a foregone conclusion - so make sure you've tested the waters and researched thoroughly.

And again this speaks to the calm and calculated nature of the warrior – the warrior does not rush in headlong, despite their control over their fear.

Chapter 38. Lessons From The Prince

Whosoever desires constant success must change his conduct with the times.

This is particularly important to note if you run a large organization and are in danger of resting on your laurels. Be thinking one step ahead at all times if you want to avoid the same fate as Kodak.

This echoes the sentiments we discussed earlier too, about being willing to *change* your principles and adapt where necessary. But this should come from within, not from without.

Men ought to be well treated or crushed, because they can avenge themselves of lighter injuries, of more serious ones they cannot.

'Crushing' your opponents and employees may not be encouraged in ethical business (interestingly Sun Tsu is actually much more pacifist than Machiavelli) but the point is still valid - don't make enemies then give them time to lick their wounds.

As far as possible, the warrior should avoid combat and confrontation. They should seek to please everyone and find the most mutually beneficial outcome.

However, if you *do* decide to engage in competition or combat, then you must act with finality.

The wise man does at once what the fool does finally.

I.e. Time is money and indecision is a recipe for failure.

Entrepreneurs are simply those who understand that there is little difference between obstacle and opportunity and can turn both to their advantage.

This is far more literal than you might think. Opening a tin of beans easily: challenge or opportunity? This is similar to the ideas we discussed earlier seeing the challenge as a chance for growth. And how crazy is it to think that Machiavelli might have had such relevant and useful advice for *modern* entrepreneurs.

Yet more proof that the warrior mindset is timeless and just as important today as ever before. Anything can be approached as a warrior.

I highly recommend reading these books as part of your evolution and your journey to becoming the best version of yourself. They belong on every warrior's reading list.

Chapter 39. Conclusion: Taking a Harder Road

We're reaching the end of our journey together now but yours is only beginning. It's time to start putting yourself out there, testing yourself, growing, taking on challenges and deciding what's important to you. It's time to stop fretting the small stuff, to cease the creature comforts and to embrace a more challenging and demanding life – because that's where the value comes from and that's what will make you great.

But a word of caution before you go: this is going to be tough.

You are going to find that sometimes, doing the right thing and ignoring your emotional response means saying things people don't like.

Sticking to your principles will mean upsetting the apple cart. Forgetting how you look will lead you to sometimes be shunned.

Forgetting physical possessions will leave you sometimes feeling destitute.

But if you know yourself truly if you know your goals, you know what you want and you know the principles you want to live by… then you will know the right things to do and you should have the strength to do them.

And that means living with the consequences.

And that is the last lesson I want to impart upon you: be willing to face the music. Be willing to put yourself out there, take risks and then face the flack that comes your way. This all follows on from the lessons on stoicism, minimalism, and fear that we have already considered. But it is highly important.

As soon as you learn that sometimes you'll get things wrong – and you accept and learn to deal with the outcome – you'll find that you become a more decisive and more efficient individual.

People who are afraid to make the wrong choice and who don't want to upset anyone will never be able to make decisions. They'll always be on the fence and they will lack conviction.

That's not you. You are a warrior and that means you need to follow your path and face the consequences as a mature adult.

You will ask for forgiveness and not permission. And if you don't get it? As long as you have done what's right *by you*, then you forge ahead anyway.

Bonus Book - Healthy yourself -

Table of Contents

Introduction

Chapter 1 – Know Thy Self

Chapter 2 – Know Thy Limits

Chapter 3 – Be Honest

Chapter 4 – Be Kind

Chapter 5 – Be Forgiving

Chapter 6 – Be Generous

Chapter 7 – Be Yourself

Conclusion

Introduction

I am so tired of all the negativity around me! Are you? This world is toxic and it is sick. I hate watching the news, reading the newspaper or even interacting with my neighbors. I don't want to appear antisocial. I genuinely love people. But this world has made us cold and cruel.

The result is a society of unhappy people. Well over 50% of all marriages end in divorce. Well over 50% of all young adults do not even believe in marriage. We need to get back to the days where it was easy to talk to strangers and it was unnatural not to be polite.

Back to the days where people actually believed in love and looked out for their neighbors. We need to start loving ourselves again. We each need to be the change we wish to see in the world. We need to heal ourselves and start loving ourselves again.

Happy people are successful people. This is simply because being happy makes it easy to stay motivated to reach your goals. Your thoughts have a very significant impact on the life you lead and the quality of the relationships you will have with family members, friends, and significant others. Some even reason that

our thoughts and beliefs can have an even stronger effect on our health than modern medicine. Consider these examples:

- A middle-aged man dies a day after his doctor diagnosed him with cancer, even though his autopsy revealed he was misdiagnosed.

- Many women who are desperate to have a child will begin to have real symptoms of pregnancy such as cravings and an increase in the size of their breasts, even though they are not pregnant.

- People who suffer from Depression who participate in clinical trials for new antidepressants start experiencing an improvement in their moods although they were given the placebo and not the actual drug.

That being said, it has been scientifically proven that you can improve your health, career, and relationships simply by improving the way you think about yourself and the world around you. This is a lot cheaper than paying for sessions with a therapist or paying a Divorce Lawyer.

This book is intended to help you heal yourself of all the scars and the influence of all the negativity around. I guarantee that learning to rid yourself of the pain of this world will drastically improve the quality of your life from this point forward.

Chapter 1 – Know Thy Self

"The more you know yourself, the more patience you have for what you see in others." - Erik Erikson

Knowing who you are is a very crucial aspect of healing yourself. How can you avoid a disaster if you are simply floating through life with no clear sense of what you stand for, and what you refuse to tolerate?

There is a reason why the small-town girl with big dreams, who gets to the big city, often ends up in some miserable and dare I say, compromising, situation.

Think too of the unhappy Doctor who is only a Doctor because his parents decided that he needed to become the first Doctor in their family. What about the hen picked mama's boy who dates a girl he cannot stand because it makes his mother happy? These three have a lot in common.

Their problem can be explained in the old saying that points out that if we do not know where we are going, any road will be the right one. And better yet, 'if we do not stand for something, we will fall for anything.' In other words, if we do not understand ourselves, this includes our hopes, dreams, and aspirations, it will be easy for just about anyone to push us into a decision we will

regret for the rest of our lives. Living down a choice you regret, especially if you have to face its consequences daily, is going to be one of the hardest things you have ever had to do.

Living with the burden of these choices is part of the reason many people are so bitter and unkind. This is not the way I want you to navigate through your life.

When we take the time to understand who we truly are, the intricacies of our personalities, we will have the keys to unlock our true potential. You cannot become your best self if you do not know what that entails. When you understand yourself, you are more likely to end up choosing a career that you love. And it is quite easy to be passionately driven to achieve great things when you are pursuing a career that you love.

Additionally, when you are at the top of your game, you will seek out the kind of partners and friends that will make you happy and thus bring out the best in you. They will understand the way you think and may very well think the same way you do too. These are the kind of people who will not laugh at your dreams or be jealous of your success. Being surrounded by loving, supportive people, will make you a kinder, happier and dare I say, a more successful person.

Individuals who have a deep understanding of themselves, are often more decisive and optimistic. That is because these individuals are in full control of their life choices and they chose

well. They are more likely to see opportunities where others see setbacks. It also takes far less effort to be productive when you enjoy what you do. Additionally, the fact that you enjoy your career will give you a competitive edge and you will not depend on the praise of others for motivation. The satisfaction of a job well done will keep you pushing forward.

I know that these may seem like ideal circumstances, where our choices are not dependent on the desires of our family and where we are all strong enough not to succumb to the pressure they will put on us to make a certain decision. But believe me, knowing and truly understanding yourself will open doors to opportunities you would have never seen coming otherwise. It will be easier for you to stand up to the pressures around you when you know without a doubt what the right decision for you will be. I am not encouraging you to shrug your responsibilities of providing for your family, I am encouraging you to understand who you are and be true to who you are at all times. You will be much happier as a result, and far easier to love, when you are not carrying the heavyweight of a bad decision around for the rest of your life.

How to Get to Know Yourself

This is easier said than done, but it is not impossible. You can start with some objective assessment. This does not mean simply asking the people around what they think of you. Your interactions with them, whether negative or positive, will prevent them from

being as objective as you need them to be. A better option would be making use of a reputable personality test. One of the popular options is the Myers-Briggs Personality type test. This test will determine which of the 16 personality types of this theory best describes who you are. It has gained popularity in recent times because its results can be used to determine the environment you work best in and even how you interact with the people around you. Plus whether you like the results or not they tend to be surprisingly accurate.

Career aptitude tests are another great option. These are designed to help you understand your skillset better and how you can use these skills to select the right career. It is never too late to start a career that you can love.

Once you have a carefully thought out plan that will allow you to care for your responsibilities and still venture into a field that you love, go for it. It might be a case that money is tight and you are already strapped for time and may not be able to make a move right now. But I would encourage you to continue preparing yourself. Keep learning all that you can about that career online or from the people around you. That way, if the opportunity should arise, you will be in a position to take it.

Once you have taken the time to learn about yourself, you may find some dirty laundry and hidden scars that you probably would have rather kept hidden. Unfortunately, you have been wearing

these scars every day in the way you interact with those around you. These scars could have made you too soft to express how you feel or too cold to care about the feelings of others. Now that you can see yourself clearly, become the best version of yourself. Love yourself. And above all else, be true to yourself. Knowing your limits is another important skill to master to navigate through this crazy world successfully. This will be discussed in the next chapter.

Chapter 2 – Know Thy Limits

"A great man is always willing to be little." — *Ralph Waldo Emerson*

A key aspect of the results of a Myers-Briggs Personality type test is the section which outlines your strengths and weakness. A lot of the mistakes we make and the problems we encounter could have been avoided altogether if we were a little more knowledgeable about our limitations. Just think about an eager weightlifter who tries to lift too much, too soon. What do you think will happen?

Any rational individual will realize that the weightlifter is going to hurt themselves. Some will argue that this illustration is encouraging us to limit ourselves, and if we do, and stop pushing ourselves, we will never know our true potential.

There is no limit to what you can achieve if you set your mind to it, and sometimes you will never know how strong you are until you try. You need to, however, ensure that reason and logic prevail when reaching out to achieve your goals. If you have never lifted 100 pounds, maybe starting with 20 pounds today would be a better idea. There is nothing wrong with thinking big, but I would encourage you to start small and work your way up. In essence, I am encouraging you to be modest in your expectations.

Modesty will not only help you to avoid setting unrealistic expectations, but it will also help you to set realistic time frames to achieve your goals. Many people become frustrated when they reach a certain age and have not achieved a certain goal. But just consider the contrast between Mark Zuckerberg and Colonel Sanders. Mark Zuckerberg founded his Facebook empire in his early twenty's, but Colonel Sanders did not become the founder of Kentucky Fried Chicken (KFC) until he was in his eighty's. Both men are considered highly successful, but each achieved success at different times.

Maybe it's just not your time or maybe you are just not in the right industry. As highlighted in chapter 1, choosing a career in a field you love, will help you to stay motivated and become successful. This theory is demonstrated in the lives of both of these men.

Their success was a result of a passion for something they loved.

A modest approach to life will also help you to avoid comparing your achievements to those of other people. Some people hit the ball out of the park on the first try, and others have to work their way up the ladder. Some will get married right out of college, others will have to wait a few years and kiss a few frogs before they find the right person. Both Mark Zuckerberg and Colonel Sanders experienced many setbacks on the way to success. You will too. Do not expect that your life will be different. No matter what you hope to achieve, you are going to have to

work harder than you have ever worked before, and you may have to wait longer than you expected too.

The beautiful quality of modesty extends far beyond becoming successful. This is a quality that will help you to stop biting off more than you can chew. You do not need to say yes to everyone. This applies both to your personal life, and at work. Don't agree to unreasonable deadlines because you want to impress your boss unless you are 100% sure you will be able to complete the task. If you have been given an assignment, and you are unsure about how to get it done, do not be afraid to ask for help. If you work a full-time job and have a family to take care of, don't commit to too much at your child's school. Know thy limits! This applies to your time, energy, emotions, and skills.

Modesty works hand in hand with honesty, the next chapter will explain you can heal yourself and improve your life using this quality as well.

Chapter 3 – Be Honest

"Honesty is the fastest way to prevent a mistake from turning into a failure." - James Altucher

The only thing worse than a liar is a thief. Liars make life difficult and often do not realize the far-reaching effects of their actions. Lying makes us unhappy people, who constantly have to be covering our tracks and watching our backs. There are few things as toxic as a liar. We should never allow the negativity in this world to force us to become dishonest people. Lying will only put you closer to the door that leads to cheating and stealing. Quit while you are ahead. Just think about the possible outcomes of a single act of dishonesty:

- Permanent damage to your reputation

- Permanent damage to your relationships

- Loss of income

- Loss of self-respect

- Permanently damaging the reputation of another individual
- Feelings of guilt

- Loss of sleep

- Loss of trust

If you research the word honesty, you find synonyms such as honor, sincerity, fairness, integrity, uprightness, virtue and truthfulness. Being honest requires more than not lying when in a difficult situation.

Being honest requires being morally upright in all things. In other words, we will try to be truthful in all things and gain the trust of those around us, using our actions. But honesty is a very tricky thing. It is hard to list all the areas in which we need to be honest.

A good rule of thumb if you are unsure if an act is honest or not, is whether you have to hide it or deceive someone into believing you did otherwise. If you will need to hide or cover your tracks after doing or saying something, you are probably not being honest.

The benefits of being honest far outweigh any challenges you may perceive as a result of this course. Think of the peace of mind of not having to rethink your every move or watching over your shoulder because you are constantly in fear of being found out. Imagine waking up and not being burdened by the heavy guilt

as a result of your actions. And don't be fooled into thinking that no one benefits from your honesty. It is very easy to become attracted to and to respect someone honest. Most employers include quality as being of the utmost importance when seeking recruits or considering a possible promotion of someone within their organization.

Being honest does not mean that we should volunteer all of our confidential affairs to everyone who is trying to pry into our business. Instead, we should not withhold relevant information from individuals who deserve a truthful answer.

Being honest also means avoiding the various means that will pop up to get more than we deserve or leading someone to believe something about ourselves that is not true. There are, however, times when some of us might find ourselves in very catastrophic situations because we are thought of as being too honest.

This is often the case when our words are not tempered with kindness. The next chapter will explore how that attribute can help us avoid a lot of the problems that can result from that sort of speech.

Chapter 4 – Be Kind

"Kindness is the language which the deaf can hear and the blind can see." - Mark Twain

Being kind means being warm, considerate, gentle and friendly. To get a friend, you must be a friend. Even more, cliché is the saying, 'birds of a feather, flock together.' If you want to attract happy, supportive people into your life, you need to be that kind of person. Why would anyone want to be around you otherwise?

As the wise Maya Angelou highlighted, long after the memory of the interaction has faded, people will remember how that interaction made them feel. When we are unkind, we make the lives of those around us much harder than it has to be. We make them feel unloved, underappreciated, and isolated when we are mean or unpleasant.

Would you want anyone to treat you that way? Would you enjoy such harsh treatment? Don't you think treating people that way at work, at school or in your own home, makes your life a lot harder than it has to be as well? Kindness fosters a spirit of cooperation, even among people who do not know each other.

Surrounding yourself with people who are willing to work alongside you is far easier than trying to conquer this world alone.

Being unkind envelopes a wide variety of actions. Our words are the most common form of unkindness. Being harsh, condescending or even abrupt, can be interpreted as unkind.

Using your words to put others down and elevate yourself is not only unkind, but it is also a very selfish act, that often causes more harm than good. A key aspect of kindness is being polite. Let us take some time to learn more about this beautiful quality.

Why Be Polite

Being polite is not as hard as some people make it seem. While it is true that being polite is becoming increasingly difficult as a result of the negative attitudes of the people around us, it is not impossible. Being polite might inflate the ego of these individuals, but our being polite is not a reflection on them.

Our being polite reflects positively on our character, come what may. Polite individuals are often thought of as kind, principled, professional and pleasant. And with this very interconnected world that we live in, you just never know who you might have insulted.

Just imagine how embarrassed you will be if you show up for a job interview, only to realize that the man you just cursed in the parking lot because you think they parked in 'your' spot, is the interviewer. Trust me, it has happened many times before and could happen to you.

Being polite involves being respectful and considerate of the needs, feelings, time, resources, values and cultural norms, of others. Being polite and kind will make you very likable and will encourage others to reciprocate your consideration. Another benefit of being polite is that it will make it very easy for you to gain the respect of those around you.

Even if they do not instantly change their behavior, they will be forced to respect you and your standards. Eventually, they may change for the better as a result of your efforts. Wouldn't life be much easier if we all had jobs in which our employees, subordinates, and colleagues, all treated us with respect?

Respect has to be earned and being polite is one of the easiest ways to earn it.

How to be Polite and Kind

1. If you have nothing kind to say, don't say it, post it on social media or even think it. Even words that are whispered to a friend have been known to turn around and bite you.

1. Don't be stingy with greetings and salutations. If you enter a room, pleasantly greet all present. When you are leavings, kindly excuse yourself. And if you are greeted, respond warmly and with a smile.
2. Do not criticize the efforts of others, especially when it is obvious that they tried very hard to accomplish a particular task. If you must offer some constructive criticism, sandwich it with some genuine commendation.

1. Be appreciative of the efforts of others. Even if what is presented is not to your liking, there is no need to make it known.

1. Try to learn a little about the cultural norms and beliefs of those around you. You do not have to share their views, you simply need to know enough not to unintentionally offend them. It is also most polite to allow them to freely express these views, without fear of being disrespected. You can always agree to disagree.

1. You do not always have to insist on things being done your way. Give someone else a chance to shine now and then.

1. Don't monopolize conversations by speaking only about yourself and your accomplishments. Show personal interest in others by asking them about themselves and listening to what they have to say.

1. When someone is speaking to you, give them your full attention. Stop walking, typing or whatever else you are doing, and make eye contact. If you are busy, politely pause, evaluate how long the conversations need to be, assure them that you

value what they have to say, and then arrange a more suitable time to continue.

Chapter 5 – Be Forgiving

"The weak can never forgive. Forgiveness is the attribute of the strong."- Gandhi

It is not easy to forgive. The very existence of the need to use the word implies that we have been hurt in some way. Forgiving a grievance, whether real or imagined, will be one of the best gifts you can give yourself. This is so whether you believe the individual deserves such kindness or not. When we refuse to forgive, we become resentful. Holding on to resentment is like drinking poison, and expecting the individual that wronged us to suffer. It can also be compared to inflicting wounds on our bodies and expecting someone else to feel the pain.

This logic is not only riddled with flaws, but it is also quite dangerous. Resentment can easily become hate and hatred is a very ugly thing. But why do we find it so hard to forgive? If forgiving someone who hurt us will be so beneficial, why does the very idea of letting go of the hurt make us feel so uneasy?

The real problem lies in the fact that none of us want to continue reliving the horror of whatever wrong was done to us. But as we continue to think about how badly we were hurt, we unconsciously begin to think about making the individual pay for what they did.

Our flawed sense of justice often compels us to believe that if we

hold on to all the pain that was caused and refuse to let it go, we will be getting the justice we deserve.

This is especially so when the individual does not appear to be sorry for what they have done. Unfortunately, we cannot force the individual to become a better person by resentfully withholding our friendship or kindness from them. We are only hurting ourselves as we force our minds to relive the pain over and over again.

While we are angrily storming through life with the heaviness of resentment in our hearts, our countenance, our speech, and our mood will be adversely affected.

Even though we may have been wronged by one or maybe a few individuals, everyone around us will begin to be affected. Resentment often causes us to be irritable, depressed, and generally very unpleasant. And to make matters worse, it is often the people we love and not the people that wronged us, who will end up suffering as a result of what took place.

The weight of resentment has also been known to affect our memory, productivity at work, ability to perform routine tasks, ability to focus, and even our sex drive. Being bitter, and refusing to forgive has also been linked to weakened immune systems, poor heart health, and even high blood pressure. As you can see, refusing to forgive will never prove beneficial.

But what exactly is forgiveness? Is it simply forgetting what took place? Does forgiveness mean we simply pretend that nothing happened? Nope. It is not that simple. When we forgive, we must involve more than our words.

We must change how we think and feel about the individual. It is as if we are allowing them to start with a clean slate all over again. You refuse to allow the situation to cause you or the parties involved to hurt you any longer. This requires a high level of emotional intelligence, self-control, and love. Forgiveness is not just "letting them off the hook" for what they did, it is allowing those involved to stop dwelling in the past and move on to more important things.

"Forgiveness means that you fill yourself with love, and you radiate that love outward. You need to refuse to hang onto the venom or hatred that was engendered by the behaviors that caused the wounds." - Wayne Dyer

Becoming that enraged as a result of someone else's actions, and allowing yourself to remain upset over what took place for an extended period, is giving the individual the keys to your happiness. It is as if you are allowing that individual to control you, and they will continue to control you until you muster up the courage needed to forgive them.

Forgiveness is also beneficial because it often results when we become aware of our faults. It becomes easier for us to forgive when we remember that we too have had to ask for forgiveness many times. Contrary to what we may believe, we are not perfect. We sometimes hurt the people around us, even the ones we love, without even realizing it. When we refuse to harbor resentment and practice forgiveness, it will be easy for those around us to forgive us when we err.

Here are a few reasons why it is beneficial to practice being forgiving:

- You will be a lot happier and in a much better mood

- You will sleep better at night

- You will not jeopardize your job by not being productive

- You will not jeopardize your relationship with your significant other or your family

- You will learn greater self-control and self-awareness

- You will enjoy greater peace

- You will gain the respect of those around you
- You will no longer feel the pain of the damage that was done

- You will experience less anxiety

- Your self-esteem will increase as you observe your strength

What Forgiveness is Not!

Being forgiving does not mean you have to be a pushover and allow yourself to be hurt over and over again. While you will let go of any grudge that you may have against the party or parties that wronged you, you certainly do not have to put yourself in a position for you to be hurt that way again. It is perfectly acceptable to be a little more cautious now that you have seen what these people are capable of. But, please be very careful. In the case of minor offenses, which are those that were not purposefully malicious, do not make the mistake of assuming that the act represents who the person is. Please remember that we all make mistakes, and we too have caused someone else pain.

Forgiveness is also not an opportunity for revenge. Declaring that you have forgiven someone is not a proclamation that you now have the "upper hand." The persons involved may have been guilty, but they certainly do not owe you anything. Even if they do not apologize, you have still gained quite a lot by extending this peace offering and letting go of the bitterness that once

consumed you. Remember that by being forgiving, you are doing yourself a favor. While they might benefit as a result of your decision, forgiving them is a gift to yourself.

How to Forgive

Because we are both aware that forgiving someone who hurt you is not easy, I would never demand that you do so instantly or all at once. You have the option of forgiving in stages. Gradually letting go of your resentment towards the individuals who have wronged you, will ensure that you have enough time to root out any trace of the bitterness you have towards them, out of your mind and heart. If you get the opportunity to see this person often, you can start by simply saying hello.

This may come as a surprise to them because they were not expecting such a kind gesture, and that might open the way for the discussion you both need to get some closure. Sometimes, even though you were wronged, it is best to take the initiative to set matters straight. Always remember how this humble act will benefit you in the long run, whether they appreciate the gesture or not.

Another simple exercise that will help us to forgive is writing down the name of the person or persons that hurt you and listing all that they have ever done to upset you. Once you have completed that list, write a list of all the occasions on which you have hurt someone, and had to ask for forgiveness. This is not something that we are inclined to think about. Seeing in black and white how often we have let our bad habits hurt those around us, especially those we love, maybe just the push we need to let go of any grudges we may have. What is even more alarming to some individuals is when they see the names of the person they resent on the list of persons who they have had to ask for forgiveness.

Another useful exercise would be to make a list of all the good things this person has done for you. This exercise will help you to remember that despite their faults, this individual or these individuals, also have many beautiful qualities as well. In the case of those closest to us, these qualities are the very reason why we loved them and kept them close in the first place. Just think, extending the olive branch of peace may even help this person to see the flaw in their thinking and change for the better. You would have made the world a better place by helping just one individual to become a better person. Such kindness does not go unnoticed or without reward.

It takes a very strong person to be forgiving. But think of how much better our lives would be if we did not walk around with the bitterness of resentment each day. Letting go of that heavy burden is one of the best ways to heal ourselves. This world was already a catastrophe, and it certainly does not need any more resentment to make it worse. The next chapter will explain how

being generous can also help us become far happier, and more successful people in this world, simply by being generous.

Chapter 6 – Be Generous

"If you can't feed a hundred people, then just feed one." —*Mother Teresa*

A generous person is not required to give all their possessions away. A generous person is also not required to allow others to push them around. Being generous involves firstly, the readiness to give or being willing to give more than is required.

Being generous takes kindness to the next level. You might be kind at heart, and often think about helping others, but unless you take the time to get the ball rolling in offering your time, energy or other resources for the benefit of another individual, you have not truly mastered the art of being generous. Generosity moves us to give of ourselves willingly, and expect nothing in return.

I know you should be wondering how giving away your assets can help you live a better life. The truth is that many often regard generosity as one of the keys to being truly happy in this miserable world. Many medical practitioners will attest to the fact that being generous is also very good for your health. Here are some of the proven benefits of giving generously:

- Reduced stress

- Lessening the likelihood of suffering from depression

- Increased sense of purpose

- Greater happiness

- Stronger families and marriages

- Less clutter

- Reduced risk of dementia

- Greater appreciation for all that you have

- More likely to benefit from the generosity of others

A generous person often seeks out opportunities to do good for others. Just think about volunteers who make their way to help out at Soup Kitchens every weekend. Those of us brave enough to sign up for the Peace Corps is also considered quite generous. But simply helping an elderly lady with her grocery bags, or stopping to allow a child to cross the road, can be considered generous. This kind of concern for others proves beneficial because it forces us to focus on the needs of others instead of on our problems. Anything that minimizes the effect of our problems, whether in our relationships or even financially, will have a direct effect on our health. Being generous protects us from all the cynicism and narcissism that makes it so hard to navigate our way through this world.

I would, however, encourage you to be cautious as you endeavor to be more generous. Be very careful about how you demonstrate your generosity. Please be especially careful when being generous to members of the opposite sex. If you are already taken, and you don't want to send the wrong impression, avoid gifts or favors that are personal. A personal gift is anything related to one's body. Perfume, for example, would be considered a personal gift.

Please also bear in mind that your safety may come into play when being generous. Many people have gotten robbed when asked by a seemingly homeless person to give some money.

Reaching into your wallet or bag, and revealing where your cash is kept, and how much cash you have, is a bad idea, no matter how needy the person may appear to be. A safer option would be to let the person know that you will return with a gift.

I would strongly suggest that you go to a secure location, one that is away from prying eyes and package everything that you would like to donate to this individual in advance.

My final word of caution is that you need to feel out the person before being too generous. Some people like spontaneity and others prefer it if you first ask them if they need your help. Even the best of intentions

can put you in awkward situations if they are not executed correctly.

We have discussed at length, how improving various aspects of your personality can help you to heal yourself, and avoid a lot of the emotional baggage that comes along with the negativity in this world. The final of this book holds the most important key to healing all the scars caused by this nasty world. Please read on to learn more about what that is.

Chapter 7 – Be Yourself

"Be yourself; everyone else is already taken." — Oscar Wilde

"The greatest gift you ever give is your honest self." — Fred Rogers

We all need to learn to be ourselves again. This is one of the most crucial aspects of successfully navigating through this catastrophe we call life. This encouragement is in no way giving you the right to be a jerk. We have already discussed that healing ourselves from the pain caused by this world requires that we work hard to get rid of our negative traits.

Traits such as being arrogant, rude, dishonest and stingy have no place in your life. When we proudly walk around with these ugly habits, we are inviting all sorts of negativity into our lives. The result of that is only more pain and disappointment. That is why I encouraged you in the very first chapter to get to know yourself.

This will better equip you to heal yourself, by learning more about your faults.

So what exactly does it mean to be yourself? It requires that you distance yourself from all the labels the world around us has imposed on us. These ugly labels come about because of the way we look, the way we dress or even the community we grew up in. There is no reason for us to allow the world around us to squeeze us into a mold that doesn't represent who we are. Just think about how liberating it would be to not have to pretend to be something you are not. This is all within reason of course. We would never want to take certain liberties that may have far-reaching effects on our personal lives, and may even jeopardize our jobs. That means that you might want to hold off on anything drastic, like dying your hair purple and green, until you find an employer that is willing to accommodate such a choice.

Here are 5 important reasons why you need to start being true to yourself:

- You will never be able to please everyone. If you constantly allow the people around you to determine who you are, you will constantly have to change what you stand for to try and make everyone happy. The only problem with this is that you will be dealing with so many conflicting demands that you will eventually end up disappointing someone. Additionally, putting yourself under this kind of pressure will leave you feeling dissatisfied in the end.

- The society around us doesn't know what it wants. The media portrays both the meek homemaker and the fierce go-getter, as the ideal woman. The society also demands that men be sensitive to the needs of the opposite sex and the dangerous bad

boy as well. Which will you be if you are simply allowing those around you to determine who you are? Whatever you decide to be, just remember that it is quite exhausting to be putting on this kind of show every day.

- You will end up making life-changing decisions based on the whims of the people around you, who will not suffer the consequences of these choices. If you decide to have a child, simply because your family thinks it's time, you will be the one to have to take care of that child! If you decide to pursue a career because your peers think you would do well in it, you will have to live with the burden of a career that you hate, forever.

- The truth always comes out. Sooner or later, people will begin to realize that you are faking. Unfortunately, as we see in the case of many celebrities, the truth often comes out in a big scandal or breakdown.

- When you are content with who you are, you will be truly happy. How can you love yourself, when you are constantly pretending to be something that you are not?

When all is said and done, you need to take control of your life if you want to see real improvements. You cannot expect different results if you are not bold enough to make drastic changes. And the time for those changes is now!

Conclusion

I hope you have benefitted from this book. By benefit, I mean that I hope you have decided to make some much need changes.

Progress may be slow at first, but you will never regret the decision to change yourself for the better. Every step, no matter how small, is a step forward, and can thus rightly be viewed as progress.

The universe has a way of rewarding the good in us and helping us to find the good in others.

By now, you should have realized that the secret to healing ourselves, and successfully navigating through the catastrophe of life, lies in our hands. Unless we acknowledge our faults, and actively work to try and improve on them, our lives will never get any better.

"As human beings, our greatness lies not so much in being able to remake the world - that is the myth of the atomic age - as in being able to remake ourselves." — Mahatma Gandhi